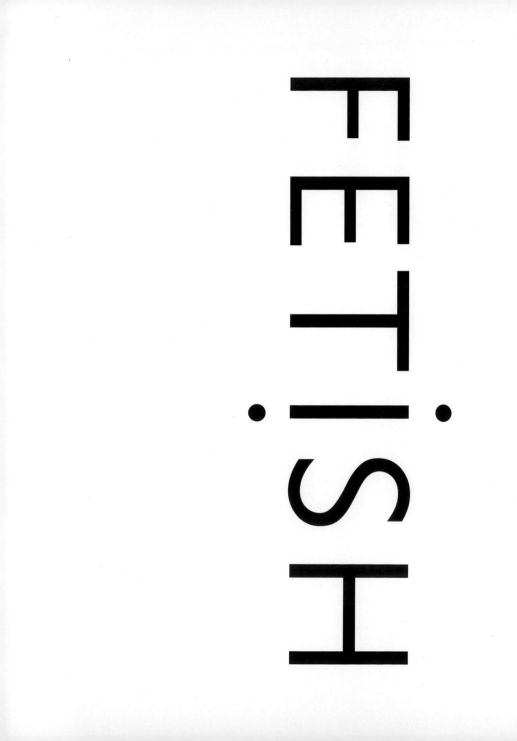

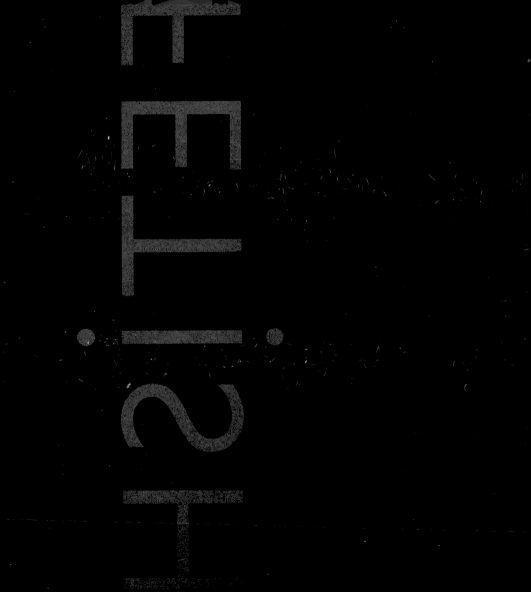

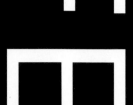
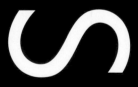

FETiSH

David Bramwell

With photos by Petra Joy

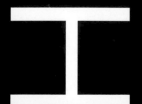

Skyhorse Publishing books may be purchased in bulk at special discounts for sales promotion, corporate gifts, fund-raising, or educational purposes. Special editions can also be created to specifications. For details, contact the Special Sales Department, Skyhorse Publishing, 307 West 36th Street, 11th Floor, New York, NY 10018 or info@skyhorsepublishing.com.

Skyhorse® and Skyhorse Publishing® are registered trademarks of Skyhorse Publishing, Inc.®, a Delaware corporation.

Design: Lindsey Johns
Illustrations: Matt Pagett

Visit our website at www.skyhorsepublishing.com.

10 9 8 7 6 5 4 3 2 1

Library of Congress Cataloging-in-Publication Data available on file
ISBN: 978-1-62087-798-2

Neither the publisher nor the author is engaged in rendering professional advice or services to the individual reader, and neither shall be liable or responsible for any loss or damage allegedly arising from any information or suggestion in this book. Anyone participating in the activities that this book discusses or suggests assumes responsibility for his or her own actions and safety, and for compliance with all applicable laws. If you have any health problems or medical conditions, or any other concerns about whether you are able to participate in any of these activities, you should take appropriate precautions. The information contained in this book cannot replace professional advice, or sound judgment and good decision making.

Printed in Hong Kong

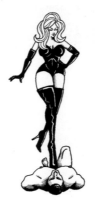

SPECIAL THANKS TO HANNAH

Contents

INTRODUCTION

Today we live in a frantic-paced world that is rapidly dispensing with age-old customs and formalities. Why write letters, visit bookstores, or bother cooking a meal when all can be achieved with the click of a mouse or simple phone call? Thanks, perhaps, to the sexual revolution of the sixties, we have even been liberated from many of the rituals of courtship in favor of promiscuity and "free love." But is sex really any better in the 21st century, or is it just more readily available? We feel an itch and we scratch it. But, like grabbing a burger on the go to quell hunger, is it really all that satisfying?

To the outsider looking in, the fetish scene can seem risible, intimidating, degrading, and even dangerous. After all, why would anyone in their right mind dress in clothes that made it hard to walk, subject themselves to a painful flogging, put their partner on a leash, or degrade themselves by licking a stranger's boots? Isn't the fetish scene just some ridiculous freak show?

And, of course, in many ways it is. But to dismiss fetishism as a gimmick or fashion is to totally miss the point; it is in fact a new and evolving erotic language. It exists outside of the everyday world of TV, junk food, piped elevator music, celebrity gossip, the intrusion of cell phones, and all that deadens our senses.

To question why a masochist likes to be beaten is to ask why a mountaineer likes to climb. Isn't it the *experience* of life many of us are seeking?

Whether through intense sadomasochistic play or scaling a mountain, it's the challenge, endurance, and sheer exhilaration of feeling alive that draws people in. And one of the many attractions of the fetish scene is that by subverting gender roles, blurring the distinction between pain and pleasure, turning violence into expressions of love, tenderness, and devotion, it transcends the duality of everyday life and allows us, for a time at least, to be someone entirely different. For others, like the destitute painter driven by passion to continue with his art despite hardship and failure, fetishism is simply a desire within that refuses to be ignored.

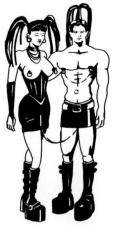

ISN'T THE FETISH SCENE JUST SOME RIDICULOUS FREAK SHOW FOR MISFITS?

Make your own rules—ignore the stereotypes and choose your own costumes and props

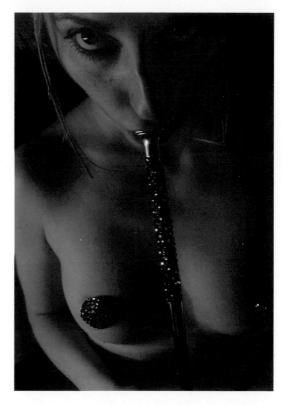

But of course the only way to truly understand the fetish world is through participation. And while sadomasochism, bondage, and discipline are intrinsic to the scene, it doesn't mean you've got to be hog-tied and beaten half to death to appreciate its value. In fact, the only really essential elements to fetish play are that it be consensual and safe. Beyond this the rules are your own: the costumes and clothes, whatever turns you on, the roles are entirely of your own devising. For some it's simply a means of bringing drama to the bedroom, for others it's a way of life. And, while certainly not precluding promiscuity and good old-fashioned intercourse, fetish role-play does demand pomp and ceremony, etiquette, diligence, and atmosphere. It isn't just about bringing ritual back into sex, but sexualizing ritual itself.

By attempting to classify fetishes, this book is trying to achieve the impossible: there are as many categories of fetishes as there are kinky people. Not only that, but the fetish scene is constantly evolving by drawing from culture. It isn't inconceivable that ten years from now Nike sneakers, lycra biking shorts, and furry Simpsons costumes may well be part of a fetishist's wardrobe.

But, while acknowledging the book's limitation, it's hoped that in the following pages the reader will find a wealth of information and advice that clarifies and celebrates a scene where the only limitations to what now constitutes eroticism, sensuality, and pleasure in the 21st century is the imagination.

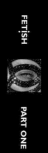

FETİSH

PART ONE

WHAT İS FETİSHİSM?

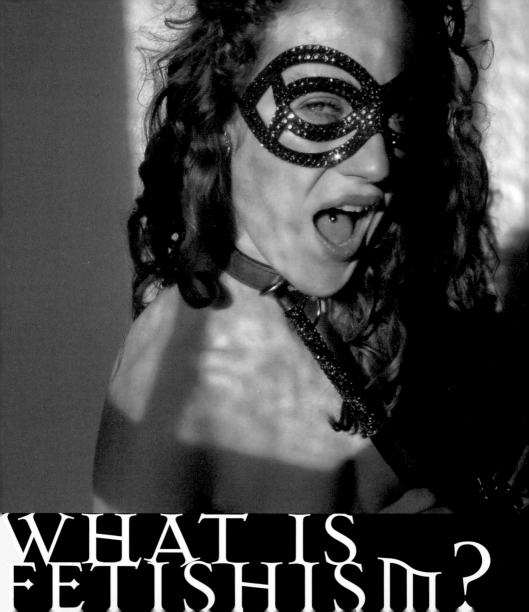

WHAT IS FETISHISM?

The word "fetish" derives from the Portuguese *feitiço*, meaning "false power." It was first used in the 15th century by European colonialists to describe the objects, charms, and dolls used as talismans by many of the African tribes they encountered.

These "fetishes," revered and worshiped by the tribes-people, were believed to have strong magical powers; an idea dismissed as superstitious nonsense by the colonialists, who viewed such practices as un-Christian.

In their eyes the Africans were worshiping false idols, and the word "fetish" became used as a term of mild ridicule.

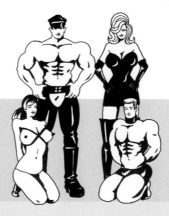

Once used to describe objects and charms, "fetish" now has very different connotations

A Brief History of Fetishism

In the late 18th century the psychiatrist Richard Freiherr von Krafft-Ebing coined the phrases "sadism" and "masochism" (S&M) to describe people who enjoyed giving or receiving pain in a sexualized context. He was also the first person to use the word "fetish" in relation to sexuality, describing it as a "hereditodegenerescene" perversion, a term which, for obvious reasons, never came into popular usage. Sadism, masochism, and fetish were, Ebing concluded, "psychological disorders" that needed to be cured.

Hot on the trail came that notorious cocaine-fiend and penis-obsessive Sigmund Freud, who defined fetish as the sexualizing of inanimate objects such as shoes and underwear. To Freud, a fetishist was someone who actually *needed* the presence of their fetish object to become aroused, and whose "disorder" had come about because of castration fantasies. Women, not needing to worry about someone running up and chopping off their penises, were excluded from the theory. In Freud's world, women simply didn't have fetishes.

From the 1970s onward, however, mainstream attitudes toward what had once been considered deviant forms of sexuality slowly began to change. Fetish fashion made its first foray in the public eye through the punk scene in the UK (and, to a lesser degree, in the United States), which embraced all things kinky, leading to the then shocking sight of teenagers wandering the streets in bondage pants, dog collars, and PVC. (Since then, from punk to grunge to goth, fetish clothing has continued to be popularized in fashion, from the catwalks to Hollywood movies.)

From the early 1980s onward, new fetish clubs began to be established in major cities around the West. Once out of the closet, the scene exploded. Nowadays, places like New York, San Francisco, London, Berlin, and Amsterdam have huge fetish scenes offering many regular monthly club nights, private parties, munches (informal S&M social gatherings), even cafés and workshops dedicated to the scene.

While, on the outside, the fetish scene may have edged closer to mainstream culture, there are still huge taboos around the subject. It may be *de rigueur* these days for models and actresses to pose with a whip or in a shiny black catsuit, but that doesn't mean there is a greater understanding or acceptance of the complex rituals and role-play at work in the fetish world. Walking down the street in rubber is still guaranteed to invite comment, and there remain huge stigmas against cross-dressing and sadomasochism. If a man is led around on a lead by a woman dressed in thigh-high boots, the common response may be "Why does he degrade himself that way?" But for many in the fetish scene, the taboo and risqué nature of these rituals is part of the appeal. Fetishism is genuinely subversive and it turns our understanding of the world on its head. In fetish play, things are different: pain is expressed as love, humiliation as respect; genders are mixed, and roles are inverted.

Fetishism is like normal sex (if in fact "normal sex" exists)—it's whatever works for you.

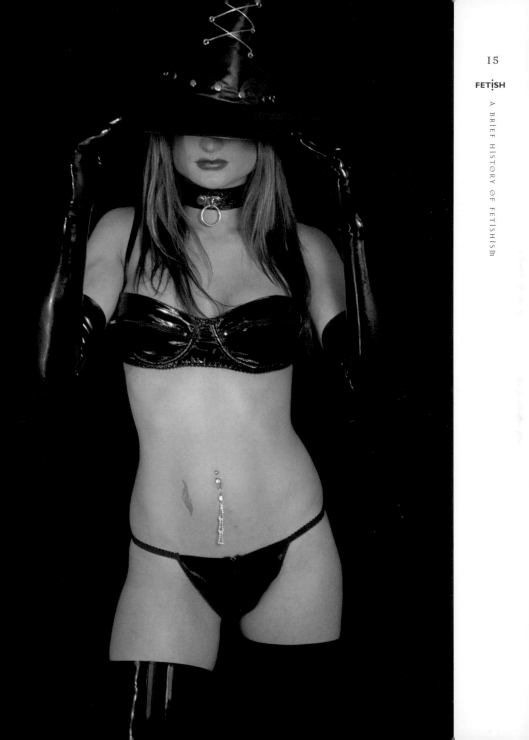

WHAT IS A FETISH?

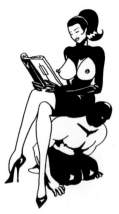

Nearly all of us have preferences for the kind of ideal partner we'd like—blond not brunette, tall not short, Democrat not Republican, sane not insane—not to mention particular likes and dislikes in the bedroom. You may prefer big breasts to small ones, fellatio over penetrative sex; enjoy the feel of satin against your skin when lovemaking, or dressing up in kinky underwear to give your partner (and yourself) a bit of a thrill. For most people these kinds of activities add excitement to bedroom games, keeping the libido alive. If, however, you regularly fantasize about ritualized erotic scenarios, or have some item you consider an essential part of your sexual play (you regularly fantasize about being dressed in leather and tied up for intercourse, for example), then this may be considered as a fetish.

While fetishism was once defined as the eroticizing of inanimate objects, such as stiletto heels, rubber, or whips, nowadays it's widely considered that pretty much anything can be fetishized. You may thrill at the touch, smell, and sight of such sensual fabrics as fur, leather, satin, latex, and PVC. You could be aroused by body hair, large breasts, piercings, or tattoos. It may be a style of dress that drives you wild: secretary in tight skirt and blouse, nurse's uniform, military attire, dominatrix (dom/domme) in rubber, furry animal costume, schoolgirl with pigtails, or yourself in lacy underwear. It could be the smell of a pair of canvas sneakers or rubber gloves, the sound of leather on silk stockings, the crack of a whip.

Perhaps you love to be flogged during sex, have a butt plug inside you, be humiliated and forced to kneel at your partner's feet while they chastise you. It may even be a specific scenario you enjoy playing out: sucking on the heel of a stiletto, being taken over a headmistress's knee and spanked, being given an enema, watching someone smoke, playing doctor and patient, master and slave, being treated as a pony, trained as a puppy, or even used as a piece of human furniture.

SHORT OF FURNITURE? A WILLING SUB
CAN MAKE AN EXCELLENT CHAIR

Since the early days of Freudian psychology, many theories have been developed in an attempt to explain fetishism. That it's linked to traumatic childhood experiences and the sexualizing of our fears remains the most common theory. Sacher-Masoch, the author of *Venus in Furs*, certainly believed that his fetish for furs and whips came as a result of a childhood incident in which he accidentally stumbled across his fur-clad aunt having a clandestine sexual encounter, and she later horsewhipped the young Sacher-Masoch for his alleged furtive voyeurism.

Other theories link fetishism to overbearing parents, or drone on about how crawling at our mother's feet as babies can lead to an eroticizing of shoes. And while theories of this kind are worthy of consideration, they all seem to be rather stark—a bit like a scientist trying to tell us that love is merely a survival instinct, the result of chemical changes in our brains. Fetishism can't be explained away any more than love, music, dance, or drama. It's a mysterious ritual, a performance, a private play between two or more people; an act of worship, both absurd and sublime. As the Hindus say, "Life is a musical; the point is to dance."

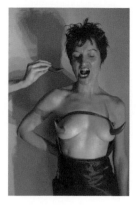

And besides, what has the image of a domme in black thigh-high boots, collar, whip, corset, and long gloves, for example, got to do with the way our mothers used to dress, or some childhood trauma? This image is much greater than just an individual experience. It's an archetypal image that comes from the same mysterious place as dreams, myths, and fantasy—the subconscious. And when you take part in a fetish ritual you re-enter that world of the subconscious and you get lost in the dance.

FAMOUS FETISHISTS

MARQUIS DE SADE
(1740–1814)

A bad boy of rock 'n' roll two hundred years before his time, de Sade has been described as libertine, misogynist, philosopher, lunatic, and, conversely, "one of the sanest men who ever lived." An aristocrat and author of scatological, amoral, and violent erotica, de Sade let his hedonistic fantasies loose upon the page. His stories involved the deflowering and abuse of women and men through anal sex, whipping, incarceration, and enforced masturbation. His most famous works include *120 Days of Sodom*, *Justine*, and *Dialogue Between a Priest and a Dying Man*.

Although he never actually committed any crime de Sade spent 29 years of his life behind bars, or in different asylums, being deemed a menace to society. He wasn't, however, without his own moral code—during the brutal and bloodthirsty revolution of 1789, when he was briefly serving as president for his region of Paris, he was thrown back in jail for refusing to carry out executions, including the beheading of his mother-in-law, a woman who had had him incarcerated for over ten years!

BETTIE PAGE
(b.1923)

She was already a famous pin-up by the late 1940s, but Bettie really came into her own in the following decade when she began working with husband-and-wife team Irvin and Paula Claw, who produced "specialist" pictures for fetish clients. It was they who were responsible for the classic kinky images of Bettie tied up and helpless like a heroine from a silent movie, Bettie as the whip-wielding domme, and Bettie in a catfight. But regardless of whether she was modeling in leopardskin on a beach, hog-tied with a ball gag, or bending a whip over her knee, one of the most endearing qualities of Bettie's celluloid persona is the sense of naughtiness she projects in every picture.

The face that launched a thousand haircuts, Bettie remains the iconic image of fetish and pin-up. Fifty years after her retirement, her black bangs, seamed stockings, whip, and mischievous face are still synonymous with glamour, naughtiness, and kink.

THE CLASSIC PIN-UP LOOK HAS A NEW HOME IN FETISH

FAMOUS

DITA VON TEESE

(b.1972)

Although no one could ever top "Our Bettie" as *the* fetish icon, Dita has certainly given her a run for her money in the past few years. With her trademark opera gloves, blood-red lips, forties hairdo, and wasp waist, this former salesgirl and strip-club dancer has succeeded in branding herself as the queen of burlesque, kink, and glamour through her effortless blending of retro sophistication with the modern fetish fashion.

In fact Von Teese is currently *the* biggest star of the fetish and pin-up world, and has appeared on the cover of every fashion magazine on the planet. She regularly tours her solo shows that incorporate everything from burlesque performance and feather dances to kinky cabaret.

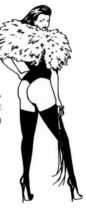

FOR SOME, WHIP-WEILDING, FUR-CLAD DOMMES ARE THE ESSENCE OF FETISH

LEOPOLD VON SACHER-MASOCH

(1836–1895)

Despite being a great journalist, man of letters, and—at one time—a potential successor to the German poet, dramatist, and philosopher Goethe, Sacher-Masoch is best known for having unwittingly given his name to the fetish for sexual submission and the desire for pain. (He was, understandably, far from happy about this, not least because Krafft-Ebing, who coined the terms "sadism" and "masochism," described them both as "pathological disorders.")

Sacher-Masoch's most famous (and semi-autobiographical) story, *Venus in Furs*, delves into his desire to have fur-clad dommes whip the hell out of him, something he actively pursued throughout his life in his relationship with his wife Wanda, and wonderfully named mistress Fanny Pistor. While his erotic fiction is dominated (excuse the pun) by theme of furs, whips, and cruel women—to the point of Sacher-Masoch becoming a bit of a bore— his influence shouldn't be underestimated. From Russ Meyer's feisty vixens to Kathy Woo's leather-clad boss in *Charlie's Angels,* we have Sacher-Masoch to thank for first venerating such feisty creatures, at whose feet any self-respecting masochist would inevitably grovel.

FETISHISTS

Safety Guidelines for S&M Play

■ Establish safe words before you begin to play.

■ Check if your playmate has any medical problems (weak heart, asthma, back pain, etc).

■ Sanitize whips if there is any possibility that skin has been broken, or the whip has come into contact with bodily fluids.

■ Sanitize all penetration toys before and after use. A condom should be used to cover dildos and other toys, especially if they're to be used on more than one person.

■ Before blindfolding someone, ensure they're not wearing contacts; permanent eye damage may result.

■ Anal penetration without adequate lubrication can cause extreme discomfort (not the erotic variety) and also serious damage.

■ Beware of constricting blood flow or pinching nerves when tying someone up.

■ Arms raised above shoulder height for more than a half hour may not get adequate circulation. Any coldness or tingling of the hands is an important warning sign that a submissive (sub) should be instructed to report immediately.

■ Take care when whipping the lower back—the kidneys are very close to the surface and easily damaged. Avoid whipping anywhere where internal organs aren't protected by bone.

■ Use extreme caution when constricting an airway such as the nose or the mouth. Leave at least one of the two open.

■ Ensure you can release a sub from bondage and/or suspension quickly in the event of an emergency. Remember, the way you tie someone should be for easy release. Don't use a knife to cut someone free if they're in trouble, as they're likely to thrash around and may hurt themselves.

■ Always ensure that play is safe, sane, and consensual.

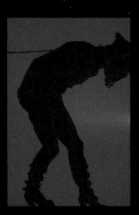

Fetish Terminology

B&D Bondage and discipline.

BDSM Bondage, discipline, sadism, and masochism.

Contract A verbal or written formal agreement between sub and dom/domme.

Dom A male dominant. Also known as a master.

Domme A female dominant. Also known as a domina or dominatrix.

Dom/me's disease Known on the scene as when "a domme gets her head stuck so far up her ass she has to have it surgically removed," i.e. is too egomaniacal.

D&S Domination and submission.

Munch A social gathering of people who are into the scene. Munches usually take place somewhere neutral, such as a bar or restaurant, with everyone dressed in their "normal" apparel.

Newbie A newcomer to the BDSM scene.

Play To take part in fetish/BDSM-related activities with a partner, or others.

Play space Any place that is regularly used for S&M games.

Power exchange The surrender of a sub's independence to his or her dom/domme.

Pro domme A professional dominatrix.

Pushy sub Also known as a greedy sub or smart-assed sub (SAM), it refers to a submissive who likes to be cocky to his or her owner in the hope of getting extra attention and/or punishment as a consequence.

RL Real life.

S&M Sadism and masochism.

The scene The whole arena of BDSM and fetish, the clubs and groups that promote it, the people who play, and the philosophy behind it.

Slave Another word for submissive, although to some it can refer specifically to a submissive who is in a long-term BDSM relationship.

SSC Stands for: Safe, Sane, and Consensual.

Sub A submissive in a relationship. Also known as the bottom or slave. This term is non-gender-specific.

Sub space A meditative and euphoric state of mind experienced by a sub when he or she gets completely lost during play.

Switch A person who enjoys playing the role of both sub and dom/domme (although not at the same time, obviously).

Training The ongoing process of teaching and learning that takes place between a slave and his or her owner.

24/7 Anyone in the scene who claims to be constantly "on" or permanently in role (although in reality this is rarely the case).

Vanilla A person who isn't into or interested in the fetish scene.

SCENARIOS & ROLE-PLAY

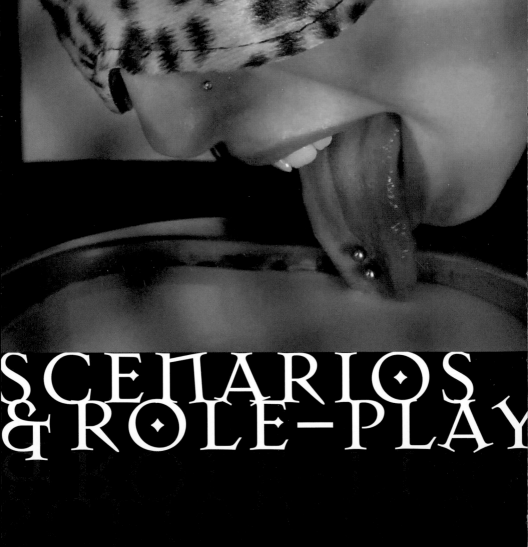

PART TWO

SCENARIOS & ROLE-PLAY

While countless couples enjoy spicing up their sex lives with blindfolds, spanking, or sexy garments, the rituals of bondage, discipline, sadism, and masochism (BDSM) role-play are often the very essence of sexual play for those in the scene.

There are many popular scenarios for fetish role-play, including schoolgirl and teacher, mistress and slave, patient and doctor, nun, ponygirl, and the ever-popular French maid. At the heart of these games lies sexual gratification through the relinquishing or control of power, leading to scenarios where a master or mistress may even take charge of something as vital as a submissive's breathing. Virtually all aspects of fetishism involve role-play to a greater or lesser degree.

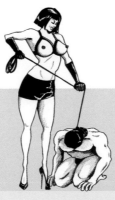

ROLE-PLAY IS ABOUT CONTROL—EITHER
HAVING IT OR RELINQUISHING IT

Owner and Slave

BDSM role-play typically involves a dominant (dom/domme) being served by his or her submissive (sub), and the two participating in erotic role-play. This can range from spontaneous empowerment in the bedroom to carefully planned scenarios involving clothes, chains, masks, boots, the hiring of a dungeon, and two dozen custard pies.

The sub, in desiring to relinquish all control and serve his or her owner, may be led around on a leash, tied up at their feet, given a whipping as "punishment," and used for sex as and when their dom/domme feels like it. This type of play can be so powerful that the sub may enter what is known as "sub space." Like the "jogger's high," this is a euphoric state brought about by a sub having surrendered him- or herself so entirely to the role that they have forgotten who they are. This trance-like and meditative state can be a welcome vacation for the mind, away from the usual personalities and roles it chooses to play in all other everyday situations, and may perhaps be *the* driving force behind fetish play.

For the dom/domme, the fun lies in wielding all of the power. They get to dress up, feel powerful in a uniform, and be the boss. Rather than playing the role as that of a cruel tyrant, however, in reality the dom/domme has a very giving role. Though the sub exists merely to serve, his or her needs will be skillfully managed by a good owner. While doms/dommes can also experience the jogger's high from getting lost in play, theirs is—arguably—a more demanding role, which might explain why, statistically, subs outnumber doms/dommes three to one!

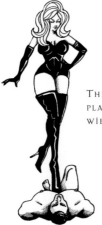

THE DOM—IN FETISH PLAY, THE DOMINANT WIELDS THE POWER

THE SUB—FOR THE SUBMISSIVE, THE THRILL COMES FROM RELINQUISHING CONTROL. AND BEING TRODDEN ON

THE ART OF BEGGING

Most forms of play between a sub and a dom/domme involve a little teasing. This can take the form of a sub being tied up with the thing they most desire placed just out of reach, or their owner taking them close to orgasm and then stopping at the crucial moment. Equally, it could be full-on chastisement. If you're a slave, how well you beg *can* make a difference as to whether your owner chooses to fulfill that desire for you. Below are a few suggestions for the novice sub needing to get into role.

BODY LANGUAGE

Put on a pleading face, sit on your hands, pout your lips, wrinkle your eyebrows, and give your owner your best "cow eyes." Alternatively, observe any child pestering their parents for something they really want, and copy what they do.

SOUNDS

There is a fine line between whining and begging. Cross it and you'll end up sounding like a maltreated dog (unless of course you're doing animal play, in which case, that's fine). A good compromise is to add a whimpering tone to your voice, but be aware that it can get irritating if overused.

WORDS

How much do you really want to wear those rubber stockings and be ridden like a horse? Tell it like it is: make promises, tell your owner how much you worship them. Try flattery: "Please, master, nothing would please me more than to have your beautiful body riding me around the bedroom."

BEGGING

Never threaten: Nothing can annoy a master or mistress more than their power being questioned. It may well break the spell of the game. If you're tied up and about to wet yourself, be honest: "Please, mistress, if I don't go to the bathroom I think I'm going to pee myself," is preferable to: "If you don't let me go to the bathroom I'm going to pee myself." After all, a mischievous dom/domme may take that as a challenge!

How to be a Good Sub

 Being a sub can take on many forms: being a sex slave, being owned, being told what to do, crawling around on hands and knees at a master or mistress's feet, being kept on a leash, feeding from a bowl, dressing as a pony and being ridden around, and, of course, being punished when naughty, rewarded when good. All of these scenarios stem from the same desire: the willing and joyful surrender of control. For a sub nothing can be more liberating than this—to step out of the "real world," relinquish responsibility, worries, everyday pressures, and hand over their life to another. But being a slave or sub is *not* a one-way exchange. It's not about being helpless, being a victim, being lazy, and expecting someone else to do everything for you; it's the eagerness to serve, to worship another, the willingness and desire to please. Submission is a ritualized role of surrender and devotion to another. And if there's one golden rule that reigns above all others in being a good sub, it's this:

STARTING POINTS

A good slave should remember all rules set up by his or her owner. He or she will do their best to uphold those rules and keep within the agreed boundaries. Some subs like to push their owners, challenge their authority or be naughty; this only works if the dom/domme is compliant in such games. If not, the sub is breaking the golden rule by putting their own needs above their owner's.

Expect nothing in return

If a dom/domme usually indulges a sub with a particular pleasure at the end of play, and one time chooses not to, this should be of no consequence to the sub. If the sub gets frustrated or annoyed, they're forgetting their sole purpose: to serve.

Pay attention to detail

A good sub should be aware of how to please a dom/domme in every way possible. If you discover that your master or mistress has a weakness for chocolates, lavish them with the finest you can find. If they've always wanted to see you dressed as a cheerleader then turn up in the costume one day. While it's important that a sub sticks to rules and does exactly as his or her owner tells them, surprises like this show that the sub has been listening, is thinking of the dom/domme, and is trying to please.

"The Desire to Serve"

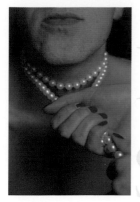

THE DESIRE TO SERVE

When in role, stay in role

Unless it's literally a life-or-death matter, no outside influences should be allowed to break the spell once both dom/domme and sub are in role. There's nothing worse than a phone ringing in the middle of play and a sub suddenly saying, "Oh crap, that's my sister calling from Detroit. Do you mind if I take it? It might be important." A good sub may inwardly kick himself or herself (and be punished) for leaving it on but, knowing their place, will ignore it. A *really* good sub wouldn't even give it a moment's thought; he or she would be too lost in servitude.

Take care of yourself

Remember, as a slave you're someone else's property and, as such, you should be well maintained. If your owner prefers a trimmer figure, longer hair, or wishes you didn't smoke, it's your duty to do your very best to fulfill these requirements. A good owner will want their slave to be fit, strong, and groomed. A mistress or master who encourages their slave to drink more, wash less, and grow a neckbeard, however, isn't worthy of being served.

Never complain or argue

Nothing will annoy a master or mistress more than a whiny slave, complaining, being demanding, or trying to tell their owner what to do. If, however, a sub is suffering in a way not conducive to play—their bound legs hurting, for example—he or she should always approach the issue in a tactful, apologetic manner. The slave should never tell their owner how to rectify the problem; that's the owner's role, not theirs. "Master, I'm sorry to bother you but I think my legs are getting pins and needles," is much better than, "You need to untie me; these restraints are hurting my legs."

How to be a Good Dom/Domme

STARTING POINTS

Communication is key in any relationship, be it with friends, lovers, playthings, subs, or slaves. To get the best out of a slave or sub, the dom/domme should find out what motivates him or her, and work with that information to create a reciprocal relationship.

Always remember that a sub or slave has chosen to give himself or herself to the dom/domme. Power exchange brings responsibility and should *not* be taken lightly; a slave who is unhappy with his or her situation will be moody and unproductive.

It takes a fine balance for a dom/domme to keep his or her slave/s happy while being fulfilled themselves, and not allowing the slave to "top from the bottom." Setting out rules before playing will therefore ensure that both dom/domme and sub have a clear idea of what is and what is not acceptable behavior. Punishment should be for punishment's sake (unless it's punishment that the slave craves; then of course it becomes a reward).

A true slave or sub who has built up a trust and respect for his or her owner will, of course, do anything that a dom/domme desires. To misuse that power will result in a loss of trust and respect, which will in turn dampen the slave's desire to serve to the best of his or her ability.

THE FIVE BASICS THAT MAKE A GOOD DOM/DOMME

- *The ability to listen*
- *The ability to empathize with someone else's desires/fantasies while retaining a clear idea of their own personality and limits*
- *Good manners and etiquette*
- *A good imagination and the ability to think on the spot*
- *The ability to laugh at oneself*

"You do not learn to become a Dominant, you just are one."

Mistress Absolute

SEPARATING THE GOOD FROM THE BAD

One of the things that separate good doms/dommes from the rest is their ability to enjoy what they do, and have fun in play. The word is "play," after all, and play is supposed to be fun.

A good dom/domme will correct mistakes in a slave's behavior when they come up. A typical mistake is how he or she is referred to. For example, a slave can be owned by a mistress, but a mistress can't be owned. So the phrase "my mistress," is inappropriate. When receiving correspondence from a slave the mistress should insist that "Mistress" is always spelled with a capital M, and when referring to "Her" or "She" the word is also capitalized, showing her importance. Likewise, "slave" should always be in small letters, and a slave should refer to himself or herself as "i."

The best doms/dommes don't need to shout or scream to get something done. A look, or click of the fingers, should be enough to direct the sub to the task in question. This sort of response to the dom/domme will come over time, and with training. It's a delight to watch when a slave is so well trained and attentive that he or she manages to serve and attend to their owner with minimum effort or obvious direction on the owner's part.

The best doms/dommes have an air about them that makes a true sub know immediately that they're a master or mistress. There are many stories of sub men being spellbound by a woman as she walks into a room and throwing themselves at her feet.

It's the fun that the dom/domme has, and his or her own sadistic style, that makes them what they are. Just being a bitch doesn't make a woman a mistress.

Every sub is different, as is every dom/domme. It's the development and discovery that a dom/domme and sub make in their relationship that can make the lifestyle so interesting.

Mistress Absolute is one of the UK's premier dominas, and an internationally renowned lifestyle and professional mistress (*www.mistressabsolute.com*). She performs at fetish events, runs *Subversion*, a successful UK fetish club (*www.clubsubversion. com*), does production for "The Skin Two Rubber Ball," (an annual fetish night in the UK), and teaches the art of BDSM at Coco de Mer, an upscale sex store in London.

COLLARING

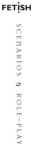

Exclusively associated with slavery and the ownership of one human by another, the collar has traditionally been (and remains) a circle of material worn tight against the throat. In the fetish world the collar is typically made of leather, metal, or rubber, and the collaring of an individual is a symbol that he or she is wholly owned by another for their sexual pleasure and/or servitude.

Some doms/dommes still like to follow the fetish tradition of using different collars to indicate the various level of commitment of the slave, from trainee to formal 24/7 slave. The practice of joint collaring is also becoming increasingly popular, indicating a devotion of both parties to each other and the S&M lifestyle. It's worth noting too that through punk, goth, and death-metal fashion, the dog collar has become increasingly accepted as a fashion accessory, and is no longer automatically indicative of the wearer being owned by another, or even being into BDSM (especially if they're sporting an "Emily Strange" T-shirt, stripy tights, and are only 13 years old).

Collaring does, of course, exist outside of the fetish arena, in the form of the tie. The ritual donning of a tie, tied tight against the throat, symbolizes the commitment or surrender of the wearer to a system, a formal ritual (such as a wedding), or simply "working for The Man." The message a businessman gives at the end of the day in loosening his tie is that of emancipation. Work has relinquished its control—for a few hours he is a free man. To talk of a priest in a collar, of course, isn't to imply he has a dominatrix for a wife, but that he is wearing it as a sign of his commitment and surrender to God.

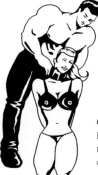

COLLARING CAN BE AN
IMPORTANT RITUAL IN FETISH
PLAY, SIGNIFYING THE MOMENT
OF SURRENDER TO ANOTHER

Medical Play

An eroticized game of doctors and nurses, medical play combines the uniforms, scenarios, and equipment commonly associated with this profession with games of power exchange, bondage, and humiliation.

One of the most popular scenarios played out by medical fetishists is the "intimate examination." This can range from a gynecological investigation by a male doctor with white coat, stethoscope, clipboard, and obligatory dandruff, to a nurse dressed in latex getting over-familiar with a male patient's rectum—taking his temperature, inducing an enema, inserting suppositories, or pretending to look for her lost pen. In other medical fetish scenarios a patient may be asked to strip in front of the doctor, given a bed bath or sponge-down from a strict nurse, be supervised in visiting the bathroom, bandaged, forced to give sexual attention to the doctor, or even subjected to (mock) surgery.

For some fetishists there is nothing more seductive than to see and feel the cold steel of surgical equipment. Stethoscopes, neuro-wheels and speculums are all highly erotic implements for some fetishists, and of course no medical examination would ever be complete without a pair of latex gloves.

It's worth bearing in mind that medical role-play does require getting into character. If exploring it with a partner for the first time, discuss your role, the kind of person your partner wants you to be (a rubber-clad, sex-crazed hillbilly nurse?), and how the power exchange is to work between the two of you.

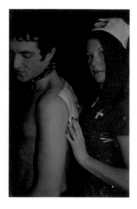

The Basics

- Nurse's outfit (genuine, rubber, PVC, etc.)
- Doctor's lab coat
- Vintage medical equipment (try looking on eBay)
- Latex gloves
- Enema or douche kits
- Bandages and band-aids
- Medical scissors
- Speculum
- Clipboard

Safety in Medical Play

- Ensure all equipment is sterilized before and after play
- Be careful not to use equipment that can cause internal tearing
- Never perform real surgery of any type on your partner

DRESSING UP

Every day we make decisions—conscious or otherwise—about what to wear. If we work in a formal environment we may be expected to wear a business suit, but if we're meeting friends in a bar we may opt for something informal and comfortable like jeans and a sweater. If we're going to a party and want to flirt we may pick an outfit that is sensual, revealing, and less comfortable than we'd normally wear (this is particularly true for women), such as a tight skirt or pants, high heels, or a low-cut shirt or dress in an attention-drawing fabric like satin. It's a cliché, but the clothes we wear often define the roles we have chosen to play in our lives.

While certain fabrics and styles prevail in the fetish world, there is no right or wrong in what to wear; it's whatever turns you on. You may love wearing tight skirts and impossibly high heels; the idea of dressing in rubber may give you a secret thrill, even though you've yet to try it. Perhaps you've always had a thing for schoolgirls, bad cops, prison guards, nurses, or even Captain Kirk. What's important is the sense of liberation that comes from dressing up for erotic games. Fetish clothing can radically transform the way the body looks, it can authenticate kinky roles, enable the wearer to feel sexy, powerful, or submissive, and be crucial in fantasies of transforming into the opposite gender. One need only visit an S&M club to witness the fantastic spectacle of rubber-clad dommes, men in military uniforms, scantily clad slaves, leather dykes, cross-dressing men in PVC skirts and heels, and even couples in full period costume.

For some couples, an important element of wearing fetish clothing is to establish power-roles in play: who's on top, who's below, who's surrendering power, who's playing the daddy? The uniform of jeans and a T-shirt is, for the most part, sexless, casual, and non-threatening. However, dress someone in the revealing attire of a rubber maid's uniform and—regardless of their sex—they'll be transformed into servitude. Alternatively, fetish clothing such as military uniforms, dominatrix attire, and leather gloves leaves no doubt as to who's in charge.

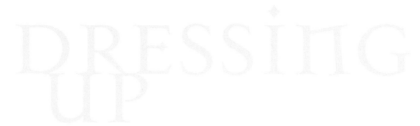

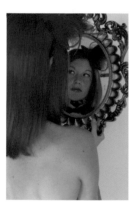

Dressing up can start small and then lead on to bigger things

That said, fetish clothing can be surprisingly versatile in the kind of message it gives out. What could be more submissive than a slave collared, corseted, and dressed in hobble skirt and five-inch heels as a symbol of enslavement, restriction, and (for men) feminization? But if this were simply the case, how could a mistress look so powerful and forbidding in exactly the same attire? The answer is that this type of fetish attire forms an impersonal barrier. The corset and skirt are worn as armor, and access to the body is restricted. The message is: Keep Out. For a mistress to dress this way is to show she is unattainable; subs dressed this way are instead unattainable to themselves.

While some people live for dressing up and, given half the chance, would happily spend their entire life donning feather boas, glittery make-up, fancy dress, fetishwear, etc., fantasy costume isn't for everyone. We all know someone who shies away from fancy-dress parties, being the center of attention, or having to pretend to be something other than "themselves." If you're keen to experiment with fetish clothing but you or your partner are a little nervous about such things, start small. Perhaps begin with a dog collar and lead, a pair of fishnets, rubber gloves, some sexy lingerie. Once you're comfortable with a gentle bit of role-play in these, it won't be long before you're dressed in a banana-yellow gimp suit with your partner dressed as Tarzan in a rubberized leotard swinging from the rafters.

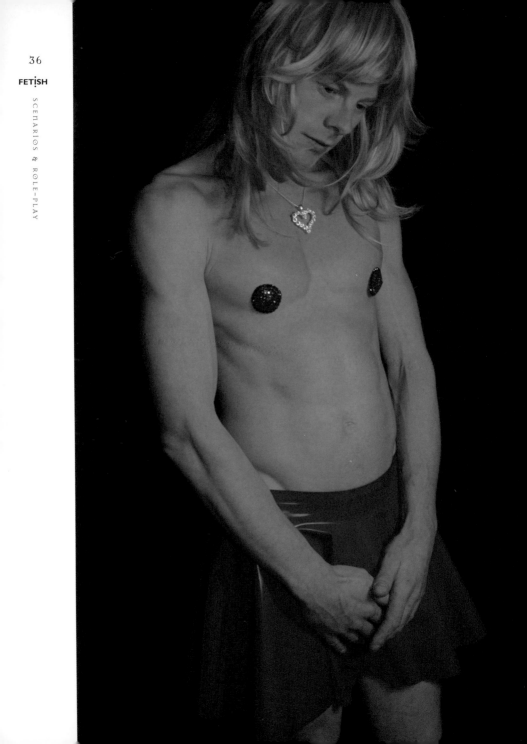

GENDER PLAY

CROSS-DRESSING

A cross-dresser is someone who, while enjoying dressing as a member of the opposite sex, doesn't necessarily mix it with any form of erotic association. Cross-dressing has a long and colorful history, from the gender confusion in Shakespearean comedies such as *Twelfth Night* and *Comedy of Errors*, to the true historical accounts of women who disguised their gender to take on masculine roles in the military. The berdache men in Native American culture dressed and played the role of females in society, even to the point of taking a husband. To associate cross-dressing exclusively with homosexuality is, however, an all too common mistake. Most male cross-dressers prefer to have female partners, but because of social constraints and taboos around men donning feminine attire, it remains relatively secretive.

TRANSVESTISM

A transvestite (or tranny), while getting a thrill from wearing female attire, may not choose to look or act feminine. In fact, one of the most famous American transvestite groups, the Cockettes—a cross-dressing cabaret troupe from the sixties—would famously dress on and off stage in vintage female attire, outrageous glittery make-up . . . and beards.

FEMINIZATION

This is the demasculinization of a man through his desire to be dressed in female attire, made up to look pretty, and act in a feminine manner.

UNDERDRESSING

This term refers to men who enjoy wearing female attire such as panties and stockings underneath their "normal" male attire.

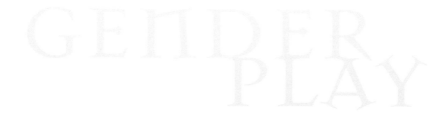

SISSIFICATION

This is an erotic game that involves the transformation of a male sub into a feminine role by a dominant female. This can be achieved with basic undergarments (bra, panties, stockings) or full attire, including dresses, skirts, blouses, uniforms, wigs, shoes, and make-up. A sissyboy desires nothing more than being trained to play a servile role such as maid (still the most popular role), schoolgirl, or secretary. "She" can also be subjected to an array of punishments (spanking, humiliation, etc.) if she doesn't play the part well enough. Sissification of a male also implies a preference for "girly" attire and behavior, such as the wearing of pink bows, frills, and lacy maids' outfits. A sissy can be used for housework, scrubbing floors, doing her mistress's hair and nails, dancing, stripping, cooking, and serving. She can also be spanked for bad behavior, and used for fantasy lesbian games.

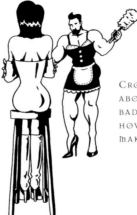

CROSS-DRESSING ISN'T ABOUT HOW GOOD OR BAD YOU LOOK BUT HOW LIBERATING IT MAKES YOU FEEL

ENFORCED FEMINIZATION

By far the most popular fantasy among cross-dressers is enforced feminization. Like sissification, it involves the demasculinization of a male sub by a dominant female, although in this game it's seen as a punishment rather than a treat (the paradox of fetish play here is that the punishment *is* the treat). The male, "forced" into women's clothes, is dressed up and made to feel sluttish; a cheap tart, who is treated and used accordingly by her owner. As with sissification, the sub may be shaved, put into provocative attire (rubber uniform, silk blouse and skirt, etc.), tied and teased, whipped for bad behavior, penetrated with a strap-on, and given "menial" tasks to perform, such as cooking and cleaning.

Owing to the demeaning female roles acted by men in this form of play, some women find enforced feminization degrading and see it as reinforcing certain stereotypes that feminists have fought so hard to dispel. It has to be remembered, however, that, as women who enjoy rape fantasies don't condone non-consensual rape, so men who enjoy enforced feminization don't view women as second-rate citizens. They're, in fact, more likely to hold them in very high regard, and hold a deep appreciation and respect for the mystery and allure of femininity in all of its guises.

Tips for the novice cross-dresser

- If you don't have a partner with whom to share your cross-dressing fantasies, find a sympathetic female friend who is willing to help with the basics, such as application of make-up, wig-wearing, and walking in heels. A lot of women find "making-up" their male friends a huge amount of fun!

- Sampler make-up kits are ideal for allowing experimentation with different hues, styles, and ideas. Don't worry if you look like a scary zombie the first few times—as any woman will confirm, getting make-up to look good takes time and effort.

- Fancy-dress and party stores are good places to find inexpensive wigs.

- Silicon breasts, padded bras, stockings, and wigs can easily be purchased from the Internet. If you know the size of your bare chest, most sellers of cross-dressing apparel can use this for calculating your bra size.

- Shoe and boot sizes can vary according to the manufacturers. If buying online, ensure that products can be returned; you don't want a pair of heels that are too tight, or to slide around in a pair that are too big.

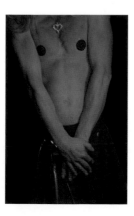

Tips on how to feminize a male partner

- Refer to his penis as a clit
- Call his anus a vagina or pussy
- Shave his legs and genitals
- Feminize his name (Steve to Stephie, Glen to Glenda, etc.)
- Make him wear your panties in public
- Refer to his nipples as breasts
- Fuck his "pussy" with a strap-on
- Remind him that once a month he needs to be unreasonable, moody, and binge on chocolate

PONY PLAY

Pony play is an erotic fantasy acted out between two or more people as trainer and his or her horse. It can range from "fooling around" at home, riding a partner naked around the bedroom, to spending thousands of dollars on bit gags, saddles, butt plugs with tails, harness, blinkers, and bridlewear. As with most fetish rituals, this type of play usually involves BDSM. Some fetishists who like to really get lost in pony play may even choose to live in a stable for a period of time.

Pony play is especially popular in countries like the US and UK where horseback riding has a long-established tradition. It also tends to be a more common fetish for submissive women than men, although there are still plenty of men who get a thrill from being the equine plaything for a mistress dressed in full riding gear and crop.

Pony play was first written about as a fetish by John Willie in *Bizarre* magazine in the 1950s, although in the Victorian period in England, live cabaret performances with girls in tassels and bells trotting around the stage like horses were clearly intended to be erotic.

One of the greatest pleasures for the submissive in pony play is to be saddled up, have their arms tied together, bit gag in the mouth, and be ridden around by their owner. In this type of play a pony can be ridden on all fours or on two legs, like a piggyback, with their arms tied behind the back. For this type of play it's more typical to find women riding men—for obvious reasons of weight difference. (If you *are* a woman who does enjoy being ridden by a man, for goodness' sake find a partner who is slight of build!)

Within the genre of pony play can also be found "cart ponies," who like to pull their owner around in a trap or chariot; "pleasure ponies," who enjoy being used for sexual gratification; and "show ponies," who take great delight in being groomed for display (there are even dressage events for human ponies across the world).

It should be made clear that animal play of this type shouldn't be confused with the desire to have sex with animals (known as bestiality). Even if someone is playing a horse 24/7, sleeping in a stable, eating carrots, and being ridden across fields by his or her master, this lifestyle remains a consensual form of fantasy role-play.

ROLE-PLAY

PONY CARE

If your pony is shaking this it usually means that it's tired and should be given some time out and a sugar lump.

Only non-verbal communication should be permitted for a well-trained pony; it's important to establish a safe gesture, such as tapping the ground twice with the foot or hand.

If riding your pony on all fours, have it protect its knees with pads.

Never use a bit gag during your very first pony-training session; it's important that verbal communication *is* permitted during the early stages. You can always pretend that he or she is Mr. Ed.

Always begin training with your pony in flat shoes rather than heels until it has mastered the walk and movements.

TO BE A GOOD PONY YOU MUST BE ABLE TO:

- *Walk properly by lifting the knees in an exaggerated manner with upper leg still perpendicular to the floor*
- *Eat an apple without using your hands*
- *Obey basic commands such as "trot," "gallop," and "backward"*
- *Toss your head around in a wild and stubborn manner.*

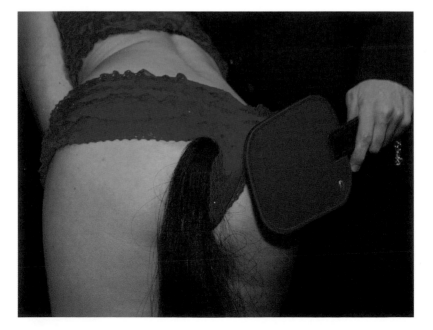

Puppy Training

This type of role-play involves a submissive acting out a canine role for a dominant owner, and it's yet another wonderful example of the endless variety of role-play games that exist in the fetish scene. While the equipment for puppy training may be less elaborate and elegant than that for pony play, there is (arguably) a more intimate relationship between humans and dogs. Puppy training offers an excellent variety of scenarios for dog and owner to act out—there are postures to adopt, signals and commands to obey, papers and slippers to be fetched, walks to be had, games to be played, toys to be chewed, and lots of opportunities for barking, whining, rolling on your back, and panting.

Many fetish puppies fantasize about being kept in a kennel or cage, fed from a bowl, put into bondage mittens to disable the use of their hands, and, of course, being kept on collar and lead. They'll even get a thrill from being taken for walk, although it's best to do this in private rather than down to the local park.

Puppy training also provides an excellent focus for games of discipline and humiliation, with the typical forms of punishment for bad behavior and rewards for good that you'd normally associate with canine training. A sub wanting to play the puppy will, almost undoubtedly, enjoy being over-zealous, energetic, eager to please, sloppy, forgetful, and clumsy—in other words, in desperate need of training. Train a sub to be a good dog, however, and, like all domestic canines, they'll be ever-loyal.

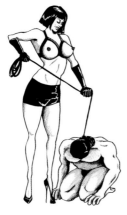

Essential commands

- *Sit*
- *Stay*
- *Come*
- *Heel*
- *Fetch*
- *Settle (this usually involves lying down at the owner's feet)*
- *Show (the dog stands at full height on their toes)*
- *Beg*
- *Lick*

Basic equipment

- *Kennel/cage*
- *Dog hood*
- *Collar and lead*
- *Gag*
- *Food and water bowl*
- *Squeaky toy*
- *Butt-plug dog tail*
- *Scooby snacks*
- *Ice cube (for wetting the nose)*

Adult Furry Sex
and Fantasy Animal Characters

People who fetishize animal characters are named Furries or Furry Fans. A Furry can be someone who likes to dress up as and act in the manner of their fantasy animal character, enjoys playing, fighting, having intercourse with fellow Furries, or simply appreciates the comic-book art of anthropomorphized animals. In fact, many Furries are quick to point out that the Furry lifestyle isn't all about sex; it's often not about sex at all. Some Furry conventions do even not allow sexualized Furry art to be displayed, on the grounds that it distracts from the purity of the art form.

The Furry fetish scene first kicked off in the late seventies via science-fiction and comic conventions, but it's through the Internet that it has really grown. Huge communities of Furries have developed online virtual worlds where fellow creatures meet, role-play, create fantasy art, and have cyber-sex.

The Furry phenomena isn't restricted to real animals; mythical animals such as werewolves and unicorns are fetishized, as are cartoon creatures such as Roger Rabbit, Wile E. Coyote, the Teenage Mutant Ninja Turtles, and, of course, all the various Disney characters from the past sixty years.

Many Furries have special costumes made, known as "zoots," in which they can get closer to their inner fantasy animal and interact with other Furries. Some have their costumes specially adapted so accessing the genitals is easy, meaning they can have sex as well as being able to go to the bathroom without having to get out of character. Cases do exist in which Furries undergo extreme forms of body modification and plastic surgery in order to get even closer to their totemic creature, although, being expensive and with unpredictable results, this remains quite rare.

A plushie (or plushophile) can be separately defined as a person with a fetish for stuffed animals or puppets. He or she usually enjoys sexual intercourse, or some other form of erotic exchange, with them: being aroused by the touch of their fur, cuddling, or using the animal like a sex toy by rubbing it against oneself to get aroused.

While the plushie's relationship with the animal may be superficial compared to that of a child and their toy, plushies often modify their "toy" to allow sexual intercourse to take place, by adding a dildo or vibrator, or creating a hole by which to penetrate the creature. Rabbits and bears are the most popular sexual companions for plushies.

SEXUAL PRACTICES

PART THREE

FETISH

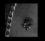 SEXUAL PRACTİCES

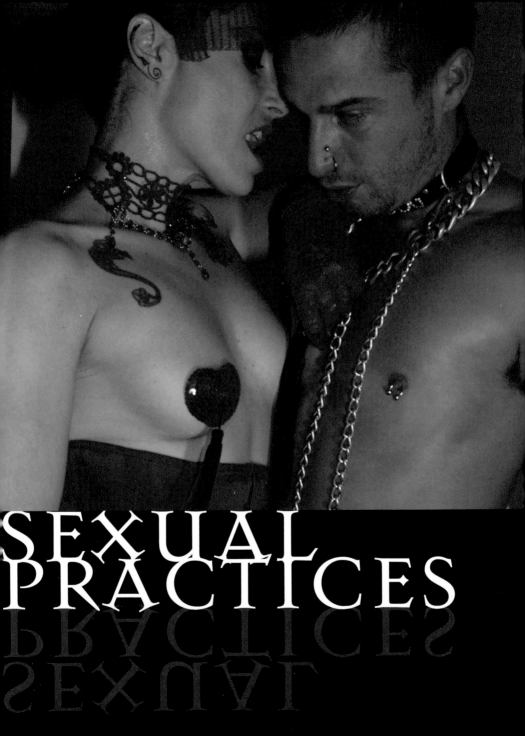

SEXUAL PRACTICES

Fetishism is a world full of costume, rules, drama, color, game-playing, excitement, emotion, and exploration.

Depending on how seriously you wish to play the game, it can even require research and study: there are special knots to be learned, the safe way to use a bullwhip, techniques for training a slave, and, of course, issues of safety. For those with a strong imagination, there need never be a dull moment.

This chapter features a wide selection of such erotic practices, as well as games that can be explored within the fetish and sadism and masochism (S&M) arena.

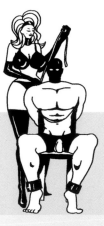

FOR PARTICIPANTS, FETISHISM
CAN BE A POWERFUL RITUAL

BONDAGE GAMES

Bondage is an essential element in many fetish games—according to a recent poll, being tied up ranks as the second most popular fantasy of men and women. There is something undeniably erotic about having someone in your power, bound, helpless, and unable to physically resist your sexual advances. Equally thrilling can be the physical and mental surrender of being restrained and allowing another person control over your physical sensations—the pleasure of release from responsibility, the switching from active to passive, allowing someone else to take the reins for a while.

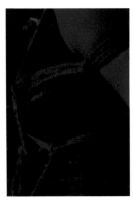

Bondage needn't just be about the physical act of restraint

Bars, cages, restraints, gags, handcuffs, harnesses, mittens, padlocks, shackles, straitjackets, hobble skirts, and plastic wrap are all part of a rich catalog of equipment available for putting someone in bondage. Rope or silk scarves can also be used (and, for some people, are preferable) as restraints. Some couples even enjoy bondage as a purely psychological game, whereby the submissive (sub) swears by a code of honor to submit to the master or mistress, even though no physical restraints are actually used. Some bondage enthusiasts may get aroused just by seeing the equipment used for bondage. Like Pavlov's dog, just the sight of handcuffs may get them dribbling with excitement.

Good bondage games necessitate a symbiotic relationship between owner and slave, where both parties derive pleasure from a game of give and take. Some bondage enthusiasts like their games to go on for hours, sometimes days. This kind of intense experience has often been compared to deep relaxation and meditative states, where both owner and slave can get so lost in play that they entirely forget their lives outside of the immediate sexual arena.

BONDAGE

Types of Bondage

SOLITARY

This is when a sub enjoys
sensory deprivation in the
form of encasement, or being
bound so that he or she is
rendered immobile and left
for relatively long periods.

Advice for the bondage novice

• *Before tying someone up, think
beforehand what you plan to
use them for and how they
would like to be used. Are you
planning on teasing them,
whipping them, having sexual
intercourse, or merely running off
with their wallet? Whatever the
case, this should have a bearing
on how and where you tie them.
If you bind a female slave's legs
together with rope but also plan
on having penetrative sex, then
this can lead to a whole lot of
trouble undoing the rope, and
play will lose its momentum. It's
worth bearing in mind, therefore,
that restraints, handcuffs, and
shackles can be removed and
replaced much more easily and
quickly than tape or rope.*

TIED AND TEASED

This is when a dominant
(dom/domme) uses restraints
to control a sub and have
them at their mercy. The sub
could be immobile on a bed,
against a wall, or at his or her
owner's feet with hands and
feet bound.

• *Remember that rope can
tighten under strain; if a sub
is tied up but wriggling
(through intercourse, pleasure,
pain, etc.), the ropes may
become so taut as to begin to
inflict unwanted pain.*

• *If you're planning on having
someone tied up for a
considerable amount of time,
then ensure they're tied in such
a way that if they fell asleep
they wouldn't do themselves
any harm—e.g. spread-eagled
on the bed rather than
standing erect.*

• *Avoid placing a submissive
partner on a hard surface
for bondage games. Tied and
teased over a table can sound
like fun, but the hardness of the
surface may soon start to inflict
unwanted pain.*

• *Learn to recognize through eye
contact if a sub in bondage is
suffering unnecessarily.*

• *Exercise extreme caution
when using piercings in
bondage games.*

• *Always apply the one-finger rule:
if you can slip one finger under
a rope, restraint, or shackle, the
bound person should be fine.
If you can't, it's too tight.*

BONDAGE

Simple Bondage Positions

HOG-TIED

This is when a sub's hands are bound behind the back and tied to the feet. While being an excellent means of rendering a sub immobile, the hog-tie still allows for them to be rolled into different positions for beatings, sex, or teasing, as they can be positioned on their side, on their front, or (for a short while at least) on their back.

SPREAD-EAGLE

This position has the sub's arms and legs spread out to form a cross. A bound sub can be attached to hooks in the wall and floor this way, or on an iron framed bed by attaching restraints to the bars of the bed. Attaching bar spreaders to the arms and ankles of your sub can have the added advantage of enabling them to be flipped over like a pancake. One of the benefits of having a sub tied spread-eagle is that he or she can be kept safely tied up for several hours in this position.

THIGH TO WRIST

A simple but effective means of restraint is the thigh to wrist, where cuffs are attached to the sub's thighs, and the wrists are attached to the thigh cuffs. A leg spreader can also be added for further control. A sub in this position can walk, kneel, and move around while remaining extremely vulnerable, but care must be taken when they're walking; if they trip, they have no means of supporting themselves from the fall.

BOXTIE

For this the arms are tied behind the back; the wrists being tied to the opposite elbows, keeping these limbs out of the way of the buttocks should a good spanking be in order.

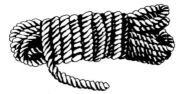

WHEN USING ROPE, ALWAYS CHECK YOU CAN SLIDE ONE FINGER BETWEEN A SUB'S FLESH AND THE ROPE TO ENSURE CIRCULATION ISN'T GOING TO BE CUT OFF

Bondage Equipment at Home

BEDS

Iron-frame beds are ideal for bondage games; restraints, ropes, etc. can be easily attached to both the head and the foot of the bed.

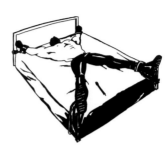

Even the humble bed can be used for bondage games

CHAIRS

Chairs offer numerous opportunities for great bondage games, the most obvious being the sub sitting on the chair, hands tied behind their back, and legs tied to the legs of the chair. In this position, a sub will feel vulnerable and their genitals will be exposed for easy access. A sub can even be restrained on all fours, facing the chair, with their arms tied to the front legs of the chair. In this position, when their master or mistress sits in the chair, the sub is in an ideal position for pleasuring their owner with their mouth. Be careful with chair play—beware of the potential danger of a chair tipping over. It's best to have the back of the chair close to a wall to avoid disaster.

DOORWAYS

Most fetish stores and websites now stock inexpensive hooks that can be fitted on top of a doorframe so that when the door is closed the hook is supported by the weight of the door and a sub can be attached to it with their arms above their head. The versatility of such devices means that a sub can be easily tied up and teased in different parts of a house, and pretty much anywhere with a door (though it's best to avoid elevators).

CEILINGS

Most houses can take the weight of a feisty slave wriggling around, suspended from the ceiling via hooks. Before you go drilling into the ceiling and dangling your partner from it, however, check that the suspending hook goes directly into something solid like the joists or supporting beams. Otherwise you may find your slave crashing back down, bringing the ceiling with them. Then who's the one who deserves to be punished?

BONDAGE

SADOMASOCHISM

S&M is a form of sexual role-play involving humiliation, pain, and control. A sadist is one who enjoys inflicting pain, while a masochist enjoys receiving pain. The word "sadomasochism" is derived from the names of Leopold von Sacher-Masoch and the Marquis de Sade, two men who devoted much of their lives to writing about and publicly discussing their sexual fantasies (see pages 18–19).

For those unfamiliar with S&M play, there are often assumptions that sadomasochists are either passive by nature, or the kind of people who enjoy hurting puppies. These prejudices are misplaced—what a sadomasochist enjoys in erotic role-play doesn't represent how they are in the "real world." Reality isn't the driving force behind S&M—far from it. While more traditional ideas of sex have revolved around the eroticizing of the naked body, in S&M it's power that is eroticized. S&M role-play between consenting adults is the gateway to exploring deep sexual fantasies, whether it be a helpless sub on the end of a lead licking his mistress's boots, or a master whipping his manacled slave.

RULES OF THE GAME

The rules of S&M vary according to who is playing. For this reason it's important that boundaries are discussed and agreed beforehand. Trust plays a vital role in S&M—if you're tied to the kitchen table with a zucchini stuck where the sun doesn't shine, you might understandably get a bit upset if your partner suddenly decides to invite the neighbors over. Equally, if you're sporting your partner's underwear in a public bar and he or she starts telling everyone, when that wasn't an agreed part of the game, this is no longer consensual role-play but *genuine* humiliation. While some people do reach a stage of "no limits" in their S&M play, for those finding their feet, the creation of no-go zones and boundaries is paramount in creating a trust which will, in time, lead to the opening of more doors and push the imagination to ever more colorful lands.

A safe word is essential for those occasions when freedom of movement is restricted

SAFE WORD

Part of the journey in S&M is to see how far you and your partner can lose yourselves. As this can often (though not always) involve the giving and receiving of pain, it's essential that all S&M role-play involves a "safe word." The safe word should be agreed beforehand, and be a word or phrase which can't be misconstrued. In role-play, "no" can sometimes mean "yes," so it's best to choose a word that has no bearing on your play, such as "walrus" or "chocolate" (unless, of course, you have a fetish for being dressed as a walrus and having chocolate smeared on your genitals, in which case you'd have to choose something else).

In other scenarios, if a sub is wearing a hood or gag, he or she may not be able to speak (which is usually the idea), so a safe gesture may be required too, such as nodding or shaking the head. But if you've got yourself trussed up so well that you can't move a muscle or speak a word . . . well, you've only got yourself to blame.

CORPORAL PUNiSHMENT

Punishment (both physical and psychological) plays an integral role in most bondage, discipline, sadism, and masochism (BDSM) scenarios. It's unusual, however, for anyone in the fetish scene to be interested in administering or receiving physical pain without some element of role-play. The giving and receiving of erotic pain is, after all, a yin–yang relationship—love as expressed through violence, pain experienced as pleasure. But if a sub only receives pleasure from a dom/domme, they're hardly taking on a subservient role.

Corporal punishment can be administered in a whole host of ways: whipping, flogging, spanking, pinching, biting, scratching, and caning. The equipment used ranges from whips, straps, paddles, clothespins, and clamps to hands, hot wax, and needles. To the outsider, unaware of the purpose of such games in the BDSM scene, this form of punishment can seem a trifle bizarre. "Isn't pain something we should try to avoid in life?" is a question that is commonly asked. The answer, of course, is "no." For without pain how would we appreciate pleasure? And besides, in S&M play, when the body feels pain through a flogging or spanking, for example, it releases opiate-like endorphins in the brain. When the body is in this state of arousal, the amount of pain it can withstand becomes much higher. When a sub is lost in role-play, pain and pleasure merge into one and the body and mind become more alive, taking the recipient into trance-like states of higher consciousness. It's really no different from those "masochistic" Swedes and Russians, jumping from hot saunas into ice-cold water and back again.

The use of pain in religion has a long and colorful history. There are countless cases of religious zealots flogging themselves into the throes of spiritual ecstasy. Recent Russian research has even proved that whipping as a form of therapy can help enormously for people suffering depression and other psychological illnesses. In fact, Tibetan monks have used this as a similar form of therapy for centuries. So remember the mantra: spare the rod, spoil the slave!

CORPORAL PUNiSHMENT TiPS

- *It's always advisable to have a "warm-up" period before administering corporal punishment.*
- *A male should have his legs closed when receiving physical punishment to avoid any accidental hitting of the genitals.*
- *The most erotically sensitive areas of the body for receiving pain are the buttocks, hands, feet, knees, and the middle of the back. Extreme care must be taken around areas where vital organs are present, however, such as the kidneys, situated at the lower back.*

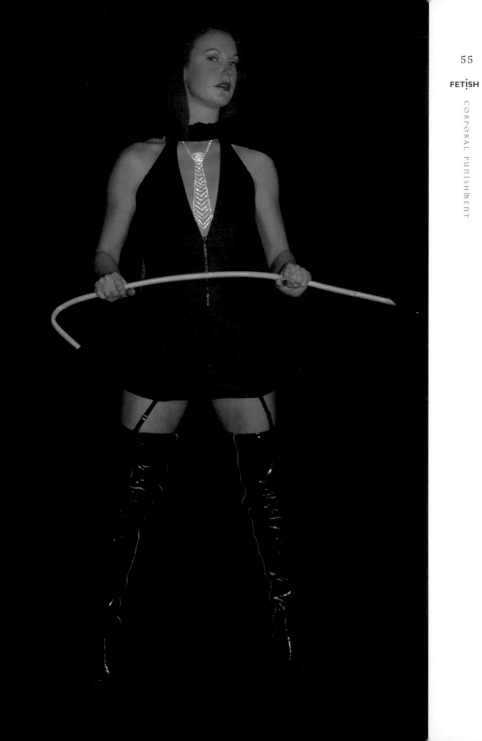

Discipline and Training

When a couple are role-playing as, say, mistress and slave, secretary and boss, or master and maid, they'll almost certainly have established rules as a means of obedience training for the sub. These can come in the form of a verbal agreement or written contract. A symbolic item such as a ring or collar can also help serve as a reminder to the sub that he or she is playing under those rules. The disciplining of a slave is of course the old, tried and tested stick-and-carrot method: punishments for misdemeanors; rewards for good behavior. Owing to the wonderful paradoxes at play in the fetish world, however, punishment (a whipping, bondage, confinement, removal of privileges, humiliation, etc.) usually means reward.

Depending on the kind of game being played between dom/domme and sub, a master or mistress may keep inventing new rules or changing old ones in order to confuse the sub, leading to inevitable rule-breaking and a suitable punishment being meted out. Equally, however, a dom/domme may prefer to train a sub until the rules become second nature; the dom/domme then takes pleasure in seeing the results of his or her psychological game, and "punishes" the slave much less as a consequence. This could involve such elements as a slave always remembering to kneel when his or her owner walks into the room, a "puppy" knowing when to heel and not forgetting that he or she cannot talk, a maid remembering to clean her owner's boots each morning, or a simple "Thank you, Mistress" from her sub every time he or she is spanked.

While humiliation plays a significant role in the disciplining of a slave, it's worth remembering that insults are best kept in the realm of fantasy. If you're playing the dom/domme, never make a derogatory comment about your sub's weight, for example, if you happen to know this is a genuinely sensitive area for him or her; it may be too close to the bone. Instead, stick to telling them they're dirty, stupid, clumsy, idle, sluttish, worm-like, and pathetic, and they'll revel and thrill at every acerbic word.

Spanking

 Spanking is the slapping of the buttocks as a means to achieve sexual arousal. It's arguably the most intimate form of flagellation in the fetish world—the classic scenario being the disciplinarian taking the miscreant over the knee, pulling down his or her pants, and letting them feel the slap of a hand against bare flesh.

It has been argued by many "spankophiles" that spanking should be considered an erotic form of play outside of BDSM. While it is true that, for some people at least, their interest in fetish starts and ends with spanking, it can't be denied that spanking plays a big part in countless BDSM role-play scenarios involving cross-dressing, discipline, and humiliation. Take the naughty schoolboy, for example, being taught a lesson by his teacher (who may even dress him as a schoolgirl as a form of humiliation, before lifting his skirt, pulling down his panties, and taking him over her knee), the domineering boss who likes to spank his secretary over the desk, or simply the mistress who wants to remind her slave who's in charge.

To maximize the pleasure/ tolerance of the recipient of the spanking, as with all forms of flagellation, it's important to first stimulate the flesh through gentle rubbing and massage, and to slowly build up the severity of the spanking by degrees.

Variations on the theme include: the recipient clothed, having his or her bare legs slapped, or the disciplinarian wearing gloves, or wielding a hairbrush.

Classic spanking positions

- Over the knee/across the lap, with pants or skirt pulled down and bare buttocks exposed
- Face down on a bed
- Bent over a chair arm, spanking bench, or table
- Bent over, trying to touch the toes

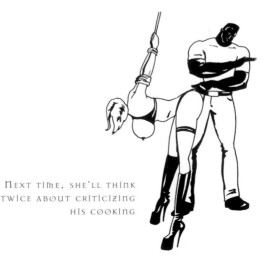

NEXT TIME, SHE'LL THINK
TWICE ABOUT CRITICIZING
HIS COOKING

Foot/Boot Worship

Whether they're in stockings, fishnets, white ankle socks, boots, heels, slippers, bare, arched, relaxed, manicured, clean, unwashed, or even a bit whiffy, feet are the undisputed champions of the fetish world. They can be licked, fondled, kissed, tickled, smelled, praised, sucked, or even used to "massage" the genitals for the delights of a "footjob." And with something like 70 percent of all foot fetishists (or podophiles) being male, it's mostly the ladies who get the pleasure of having their toes and ankles pampered and admired, usually by a fawning sub, kneeling at their feet.

To many people there is something irresistible about the contours of the foot, the smell of a gym shoe, a leg inside a leather riding boot, a foot in silk stockings, the way a high heel elevates the body, or painted toenails poking out of a pair of stilettos. And the seminal image of a leather-clad dominatrix in fishnets and thigh-high boots can have the power to make many a good podophile tremble at the knees.

While we probably all know women who claim to have a "shoe fetish"—i.e. they've got over fifty pairs of shoes and boots and still want more—there is a distinction between a fetish and rampant consumerism (Imelda Marcos being a prime example). As with other forms of erotic objectification, a true foot/shoe fetishist will be sexually aroused by the sight of a pair of heels or the smell of a foot, in the same way that another person may be

turned on by the sight of a pair of breasts or an attractive male torso. He or she may also be aroused by wearing specific shoes or boots. This is equally true of both men and women; a male footwear fetishist can get a huge thrill from wearing ladies' high-heeled boots, although this doesn't mean assumptions can be made about other aspects of his sexuality.

Traditionally, prostration before another person has always symbolized surrender; and the washing, kissing, and worshipping of feet/boots is a rich part of the ritual of submission to another. A sub may desire nothing more than to prove their lowly status by kissing their owner's feet, licking the dirt from their boots, or being led around on a chain so that the world is experienced from the level of their master's or mistress's feet.

Fun games for footwear fetishists

- *Shoeshine boy and madame*
- *Enforced fellatio with the stiletto heel*
- *Chaining of a sub's neck to the foot or boot*
- *Foot massage or foot bath*
- *Cleaning the boot/shoe/foot with the tongue*
- *Eating dinner off the foot/boot*
- *Masturbation by rubbing the foot/boot/stiletto against the genitals*

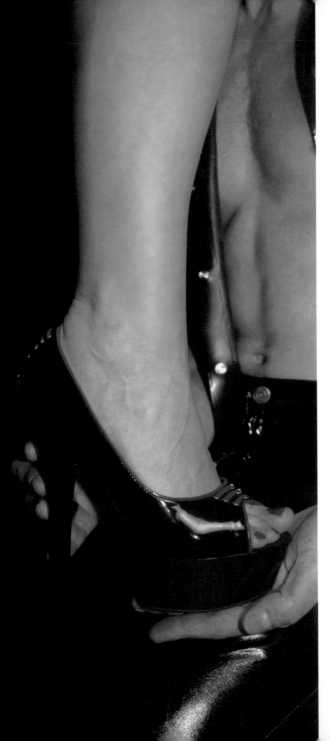

The importance of the high heel in fetishism is a relatively recent one compared to the foot. An early style of high-heeled shoe was first imported to a US brothel in the 1850s by a French prostitute. It proved so popular (clients kept asking for the "lady in the shoes") that more were imported and before long a fashion for high heels had taken off.

The stiletto heel is, of course, a powerful symbol. To a submissive male it can represent a weapon (the eye-watering image of a stiletto heel pressed into the testicle); to an ardent feminist it may represent a restriction of female freedom; to another person it could be a status of power and eroticism. When the writer and feminist Germaine Greer wrote of a colleague who wore "fuck me shoes," it's not hard to imagine the kind of style she was referring to. And if you're a foot fetishist, take cheer, you're in excellent company. Famous podophiles include Casanova, Thomas Hardy, and F. Scott Fitzgerald.

Orgasm Denial and Teasing

When French author Gustave Flaubert wrote, "Anticipation is the most reliable form of pleasure," he may well have been thinking about this particular sexual paradigm. After all, his demise did come about through syphilis.

Usually practiced as part of a more complex BDSM game between consenting partners, orgasm denial can be set up through verbal contract or the use of a chastity belt. Some chastity belts even prevent male wearers from getting an erection, forcing them to be careful to keep their thoughts pure. In many ways orgasm denial highlights one of the major differences between BDSM and vanilla sex. With vanilla sex, orgasm may be prolonged through foreplay and teasing, but for most people it's the inevitable and desired conclusion of intercourse. In BDSM, ritual and role-play take precedence, and many forms of fetish-related play don't necessarily result in orgasm.

Teasing can come in many forms. Once a sub is restrained, he or she can be teased to your heart's content through gentle caressing of the genitals, leading them close to orgasm, then stopping. Some doms/ dommes prefer the visual side of teasing. Try tying up a sub and making them watch while you masturbate, or taunt them by explaining in detail what you know they'd like you to be doing to them.

TEASING

Wax and Flame Play

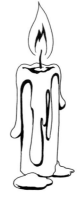

Wax play is the technique of dripping hot wax from a candle onto a partner's flesh as a means of sexual arousal. It's often performed with a partner tied naked to a bed, or on all fours, or upright against a wall, heightening the psychological effect of surrender, suspense, teasing, and pain/pleasure.

While the back and buttocks are popular areas for wax play, it can be dripped to form spots over most of the body, used to make small puddles in certain areas such as the anus, or even held over one area to create a mound.

Flame play can be combined or performed separately, and involves the teasing and mild scalding of the flesh by waving the flame over or under the skin.

Tips for flame play

- Be extremely careful if holding flames around the genitals; these areas are much more sensitive than other parts of the body, and hair is flammable.
- Before trying flame play on a partner, experiment on yourself to gauge the intensity of the heat of the flame.
- Never use flame play on or around the face.
- Keep ice on hand in case of injury.

Tips for wax play

- Use a non-scented, uncolored candle.
- Dripping wax onto areas covered with hair can prove difficult to remove afterward; the same applies to clothes and bed linen.
- The farther away the candle is held from the flesh, the longer the wax has to cool before it reaches the body, making for an easy method of heat control on the skin.

- Before dripping wax on a partner, try it on yourself to gauge the heat.
- Applying oil before wax play can make it easier to remove the wax afterward.
- Avoid dripping the wax close to the face.

Looners and Inflatables

This is a fetish associated with all things that can be pumped up or deflated. Adherents can be roughly sub-divided into inflators, deflators, or poppers. While inflatophiles get aroused from having their favorite object (an air mat, beach ball, etc.) inflated while they lie on top of it, the deflator gets sexual pleasure from the exact opposite.

The popper, meanwhile (yes, you guessed it), gets his or her thrills from an inflatable being punctured. In sexual play this is often set up as a surprise, with the popper laid or sitting in a position where they can't see their partner and therefore don't know when he or she is going to burst the inflatable.

In some instances the bursting of an inflatable can lead to the popper receiving an instantaneous orgasm without even the need for touching himself or herself. Those who specifically derive pleasure from the blowing up, deflating, or bursting of balloons are often referred to collectively as looners.

Whether a looner's object of desire is a swimming-pool toy, air mat, swim ring, or balloon, it's considered by some that the fetishizing of these objects comes from the marrying of a happy childhood experience with an intense first sexual experience. Other theories suggest that the malleability of an object like a rubber balloon is highly suggestive of flesh, leading to its objectification. Manufacturers have, however, yet to cash in on this fetish, and, as yet, the self-deflating or exploding rubber doll is more likely to come from over-use than by design.

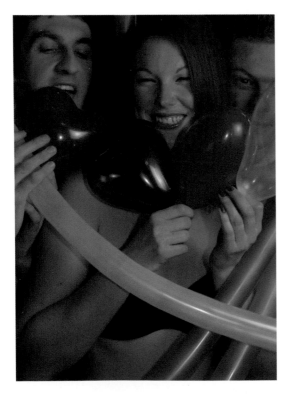

ROPE PLAY

 While in most countries rope play remains largely another means of restraining or immobilizing a sub, in Japan it has been celebrated as an erotic art form for over a century. Japanese rope play is known as *kinbaku* (and, more commonly, although incorrectly, as *shibari*), which means "beautiful bondage," and indeed one of the key elements in this ritual is the aesthetics of the (often) complex patterns created across the body by the ropes.

Long lengths of rope and a whole system of complicated knots are traditionally used in rope play. In Japan, shorter pieces, usually 23–26 feet long, are applied, and often just a handful of knots, however complex the patterning may be.

Kinbaku isn't about inflicting pain through restraint—quite the opposite. If performed correctly it can be a highly sensual experience for the sub, with the body being gently massaged by the ropes, particularly if it's suspended in the air. One of the great skills of a rope bondage practitioner is, therefore, the careful way they use the ropes to distribute pressure around the body, and massage certain parts of the body—such as breasts, genitals, or buttocks.

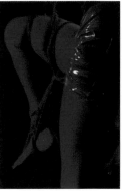

TIPS FOR ROPE BONDAGE ENTHUSIASTS

• For general rope play at home, good-quality nylon or polypropylene is best. If you're interested in learning about Japanese rope bondage, however, hemp or jute are recommended; some styles of kainbaku require a high degree of friction from the rope, and these materials are usually more coarse.

• Rope bondage is a highly skilled art form and can be very dangerous if practiced incorrectly. Good books are available for building up skills in rope play, although ideally it's best to seek out workshops in big cities to learn firsthand how to practice this beautiful art form.

STRAP-ON SEX

Strap-on sex is sexual intercourse involving a dildo or vibrator attached to the wearer's waist, groin, or thigh. If you think the pleasures of the strap-on are restricted to lesbian couples, think again.

Research shows that sales of strap-ons are now higher among heterosexual couples. "Straight" men and women have finally come around to the pleasures of pegging (anal penetration).

The popularity of the strap-on has, consequently, brought a reversal of roles to the bedroom, even for couples who don't consider themselves into fetish or role-play. With a strap-on the woman is no longer the one traditionally being "made love to," but instead gets to experience the pleasure of penetrating her partner. The man, conversely, gets to experience being penetrated by a partner, and may also potentially achieve a different kind of orgasm.

Nearly all positions manageable in conventional intercourse can be achieved with strap-ons, along with a few that aren't, such as a man being able to double-penetrate a female partner, or both partners penetrating each other at the same time. In fetish role-play the strap-on is most commonly used for anal penetration of a man by a woman, and is usually associated with scenarios of empowerment and surrender. For a man to be tied, flogged, and pentrated by a woman wearing a strap-on can be the ultimate in surrender to her superior power in the game.

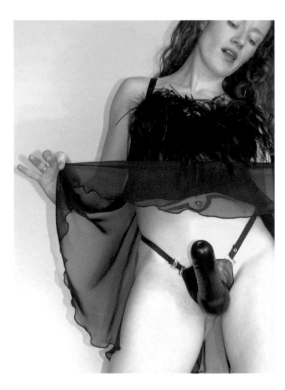

COCK AND BALL TORTURE

Though it might sound far from appealing, cock and ball torture (CBT) is a popular practice among fetishists. Being an area of great sensitivity as well as a focal point for physical pleasure, men's genitals are a prime target for games involving pain and submission. Most men will feel extremely vulnerable when their "best friend" is being abused, hence the strong psychological effect of CBT.

Different CBT techniques include scratching, flicking, squeezing, electrocuting, subjecting the genitals to temperature extremes, hanging weights, tying elastic bands, and using a miniature flogger.

Clothespins, clamps, and other toys that pinch the skin can be attached to both the penis and testicles to cause heightened pleasure/pain. Creating pressure in the testicles can also be incredibly stimulating, and can be achieved either through squeezing or by tying a cock-and-ball divider around the genitals, which applies pressure by forcing the testicles apart.

Of course, it should go without saying that these games aren't for novices or the squeamish. While some men enjoy extreme acts of violence in CBT, such as stamping a stiletto into the testicles (my eyes are watering even at the thought), it's important to remember that testicles are an extremely delicate and sensitive part of the male anatomy. This kind of play *can* lead to permanent damage, infertility, and a funny walk. CBT is a game to be played with trust, care, and extreme caution.

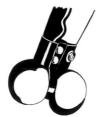

COCK AND BALL TORTURE—A MOUTH-WATERING PROSPECT TO SOME, EYE-WATERING TO OTHERS

TORTURE

OUT ON LOCATION

FETISH

PART FOUR

FETISH

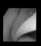 OUT ON LOCATION

- PART FOUR

OUT ON
LOCATION

As important as what you do with your fetish, can be *where* you do it. You may have a fantasy that involves a dungeon, a medical waiting room, pony play in a stable, being made to cross-dress in a lingerie department, or even crawling up inside a giant shoe and being squashed by an enormous foot.

You might be perfectly content playing in the bedroom, but perhaps you have always dreamed of having your partner in a cage at the foot of the bed, or yourself suspended from the ceiling. In this chapter, popular role-play scenarios are explored together with helpful suggestions and tips on how to realize such location-specific fantasies.

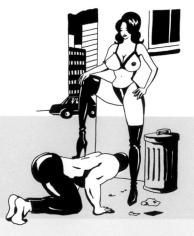

AS REAL ESTATE AGENTS KNOW,
LOCATION IS EVERYTHING

Setting the Scene

Fetish involves ritual, whether that means dressing up in a favorite uniform and enslaving your partner, submitting to an erotic and humiliating medical examination, or having a tail strapped to your buttocks and being made to bark like a dog. And to add potency to an erotic ritual, creating the right atmosphere is crucial, particularly if you and your partner want to keep in role and really get lost in fantasy play.

Setting the scene for fetish role-play doesn't have to mean building an extension to the house and converting it into a medical laboratory, school room, or dungeon (though that's not to be discouraged!); little touches can be enough.

Tips for setting the scene

- *Ensure you're not going to be disturbed by visitors, pets, or children.*
- *Switch off cell phones and answering machines.*
- *If you've set aside time in the evening to play, candlelight can create a far more evocative atmosphere than electric lighting.*
- *Plan ahead: get props and costumes ready, polish those rubber gloves, make sure sex toys have been cleaned, and anything in the room that might be a hindrance or distraction has been hidden away.*
- *Make sure the space is sufficiently warm, especially if one of you is going to be naked or tied up.*
- *Choose a soundtrack that will help to create the right mood: instrumental music may be more appropriate and evocative than a compilation of your favorite songs, for example.*

Think about what to wear and when you're going to wear it. If you're playing a dom/domme, babysitter, or even werewolf for the night, it may be far better to make a dramatic entrance once fully attired, rather than dressing in front of your partner (unless dressing each other is part of the ritual).

It pays to have a fairly defined moment for the transformation from the world of vanilla to fetish. If you're playing puppy and trainer, play might begin when the puppy hears the familiar rattle of the chain, signifying he or she is required to get into role. If you're playing the dom/domme, don't forget that your sub can always be bound and blindfolded at any time (they won't complain!) to allow time for you to prepare properly.

If you're planning a medical examination of your partner you could put new white sheets on the bed, cover the bedside table with a white cloth, and leave a clipboard nearby. If you're re-enacting one of the scenes from the film *Secretary*, clear a table, maybe put a few hooks on the floor by the table legs, and hide a flogger in the table drawer.

And finally, remember it's meant to be fun. Never put too many demands on someone if they're not in the mood. There will always be times when an eager sub prepares a surprise for their owner only to find them walking through the front door after a long day at work and too tired to play. If this kind of thing happens, don't worry—give your partner space, take them away from the fetish setting, and let them unwind. Once they've had a drink or a rest they may well be teased back into their kinky role.

FETISH CLUBS

Clubs and private parties are ideal for indulging in open fetish role-play, provided you're prepared for the exhibitionistic nature of such places. Kinky clubs nearly always include play equipment such as stocks, benches, cages, etc., and offer the chance for fetishists to interact with each other in an intimate, erotic, or just social way.

HOTEL ROOMS

There is something wonderfully seedy about hiring a hotel room for the sole purpose of sex—particularly if you've got a suitcase stuffed full of toys, clothes, and equipment in your hand. And using a neutral space such as this can add frisson and excitement not possible in an over-familiar home environment.

IF YOU DON'T FEEL COMFORTABLE ARRIVING AT A CLUB DRESSED IN FULL FETISH GEAR, REMEMBER YOU CAN ALWAYS CHANGE INSIDE INSTEAD

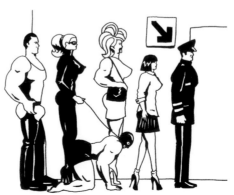

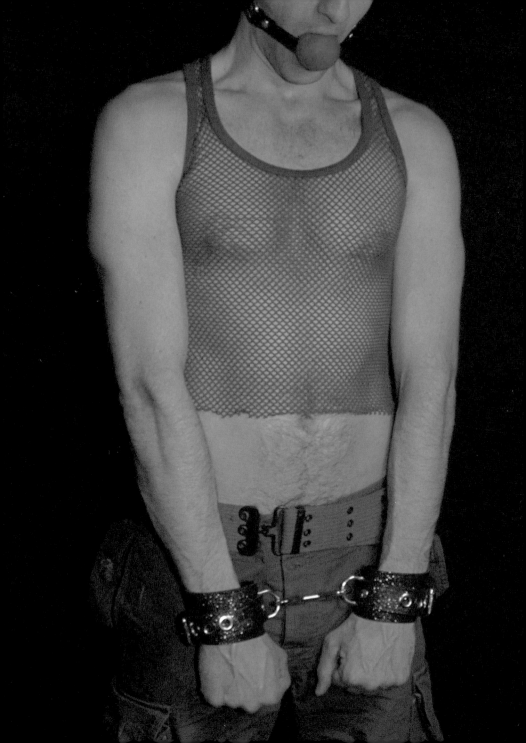

IN THE DUNGEON

The dungeon is, perhaps, the fetishist's favorite playground. It provides an intimate and private space in which couples can lose themselves in their fantasies and experiment with fetish equipment they either can't afford or don't have room for at home. A professional dungeon is usually dark, windowless, and with subdued lighting to create a conducive atmosphere for prolonged role-play. It will usually include items such as cages, stocks, suspension hooks in the ceiling, torture racks, mirrors, spanking benches, and even a stereo to enable you to chose your own kinky soundtrack.

Dungeons can be found in most large cities these days, and hired out for anything from an hour upward. Some places even offer a B&B service allowing couples to stay in role for days at a time.

If you're lucky enough to have a spare room or basement in the house, with a little money and imagination this could be turned into your own private dungeon—or at least a special place reserved for fetish play. For those unable to afford such luxuries, there are, however, more modest means of utilizing other parts of the house as discreet play areas.

An empty wardrobe is a good starting point. With a few well-placed hooks inside the wardrobe and on the back of the door, whips, chains, collars, etc. can all be strategically placed, clothes can be properly hung, and, if it's big enough, a slave can even be tied up inside among all the fetish-wear and paraphernalia. You may also want to put a lock on the wardrobe to keep out nosy visitors (or family!). A lock can also double up as a means of keeping control over a sub, only allowing them access as and when the dom/domme desires.

Hooks (or holes for hooks) can be discreetly placed on walls in any part of the house and hidden by picture frames when not in use. They can also be fitted into the floor and hidden by sofas, chairs, and heavy rugs.

Metal-framed beds, chairs, and/or even a chaise longue can be used as part of play; no one need know their darker purpose.

A closet under the stairs can be converted into a kennel or area of confinement for naughty subs.

Drawers on wheels can be utilized for storing fetish equipment and kept under the bed for easy access.

Rooms can be soundproofed to avoid the embarrassment of neighbors coming around at two in the morning concerned about all the screams.

Specially made bondage cages are available from fetish stores, and they're specially designed to be folded up and stored away.

Massage tables may be utilized for gynecological examinations and medical-related play.

WATCHING ME, WATCHING YOU

While much could be said about Peeping Toms, flashers, mooning fratboys, and seedy men in raincoats who rub themselves up against you on the subway, this book is concerned only with consensual forms of sexuality. The fetishes featured in this section are confined to examples where both parties are fully aware of the role-play involved.

EXHIBITIONISM AND VOYEURISM

While an exhibitionist craves an audience to observe his or her sexual antics, a voyeur is aroused through passive observance of sexual acts, and as such these two fetishes complement each other like toast and marmalade. As a form of play between partners, exhibitionism and voyeurism can take the form of a striptease with an audience of one, a peepshow-style masturbation scene, or that age-old game of "I'll show you mine if you show me yours." The voyeur may also prefer to be tied to a chair, filming or photographing "the show," or even furtively watching through a keyhole.

In the fetish scene, play parties are often organized for people who like to indulge in exhibitionism and voyeurism; usually as a part of other kinky games such as bondage, or sadism and masochism (S&M). These are normally held in private; fetish clubs are restricted by laws regarding sexual conduct at public events. Outside of the fetish scene, swingers' clubs and orgies can be ideal for watching and being watched, although it always pays to visit strictly as an observer first, to see if you like the crowd and the ambience. It goes without saying that rules of consensual and safe sex are of prime importance with this kind of scene.

PUBLIC PLAY

For many couples, sex in public places is a huge turn-on. While the thrill of potentially getting discovered plays a big role in this form of play, it's important to remember that not everyone wants to stumble over naked bodies writhing around in their local Wal-Mart. A degree of discretion is needed, so more realistic (though still illegal) places to indulge this fetish may be a quiet corner of a public park, a secluded beach, in the woods, or in public restrooms. Of course, you could end up spending the night in a police cell, but then this too may serve as a perfect spot to continue your illicit activities ...

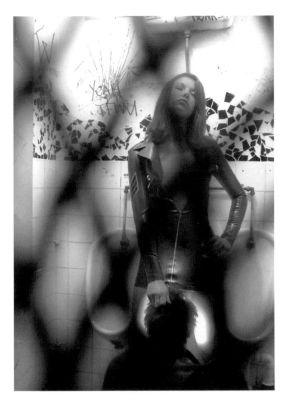

If you choose to go
public, remember
that people may be
watching, whether you
know it or not . . .

PUBLIC HUMILIATION

If you've ever walked into your favorite clothes store to buy some new underwear and been surprised to see a man on his hands and knees crawling to the cash desk with a pair of panties in his mouth while his girlfriend gives him a playful kick and tells him to hurry up, chances are the two are indulging in a little public humiliation. As well as demanding balls of steel, this kind of role-play can equally cause offence; whereas in fetish clubs this kind of behavior is more acceptable and even encouraged. More subtle public games are, however, often played between couples—such as a sub being required to go out wearing an article of clothing from his mistress's wardrobe, or a female slave, on a visit to her parents, being required by her master to wear the new butt plug he just bought her.

DOGGING

This is a spectator sport based on watching consenting couples having sex in parked automobiles. While almost exclusively a nocturnal practice, participants' choice of location can range from isolated country roads to busy city parking lots. According to some codes of practice, if the light is left on in the automobile the couple are happy to be watched; if it's off, they'd rather be left alone (which, of course, does beg the question why are they there in the first place?). Dogging originated in the UK, where several celebrities have been caught in high-profile and very public sex scandals. But such is the growing popularity of this sexual practice that it has become prevalent in the US, and unofficially adopted as a national sport in Germany.

Messy Play

Also known as sploshing, or wet and messy (W&M), this is the term for fetishists who are aroused by sticky, wet, messy, or oily substances being applied to naked or clothed bodies. Sploshing can include showering fully clothed, mud-wrestling, rubbing food into a partner's body, sliding around naked in oil and lotions, or even indulging in food fights. It's also top-class entertainment.

After all, what could be more liberating than writhing around fully clothed in chocolate sauce? What better way of dissolving an argument with a partner than shoving a custard pie in his or her face? And what could be more erotic than seeing a pair of naked buttocks squelch on a cream cake?

WAMers tend, on the whole, not to be interested in power games. The thrill here the sight and physical experience of soft, viscous food on the body, tight wet clothing, and mess in general (though sploshing can be combined with games of S&M, such as a sub having his or her dinner smeared on a dom's/domme's boots and being made to lick it off). Equally, the inclusion of body fluids in play is rarely part of a WAMer's fantasy.

GOOD PLACES TO GET MESS IN THE HOME

Bathroom

The bathroom is by far the most sensible place to play if you're going to be dressed as a cowboy, showered in water, and smeared in maple syrup.

Bedroom

If you enjoy writhing around naked with your partner in oil or lotions, the bedroom is an ideal location. It pays to buy a rubber or PVC sheet for the bed. Not only will this avoid staining the bedding, it also makes the perfect surface on which to slide around.

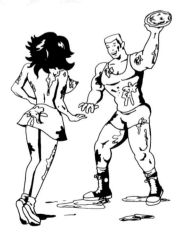

WETLOOK/WETPLAY

Clothing can also play an important role in messy play; for some, the sight or feel of wet clothing can offer a similar thrill to that of a rubber fetishist who takes pleasure from a tight, shiny second skin highlighting the contours of the body.

Wetlook fetishists are often aroused by watching other people swimming, or showering fully clothed. They may prefer a voyeuristic approach, or enjoy intimate sexual acts while fully clothed in water. Good places outside the house to enjoy wetlook sex include secluded waterfalls, rivers, beaches, lakes, and ponds, although extreme care must be taken if there are tides present. Public swimming pools and nudist beaches aren't appropriate places for this kind of activity.

ADVICE FOR WAMERS

While most natural food substances are suitable for use on the body, man-made oils or processed food can potentially cause irritation or rashes through their contact with genital areas or orifices.

Think your W&M plans through first. Do you think that wrestling your partner into the bath and pouring chocolate sauce over them after a busy day at the office is really such a good idea? Many food substances can ruin clothing or, at the very least, lead to an expensive dry-cleaning bill. Why not put aside special clothes for sploshing, or only use those that you won't mind throwing away should they be ruined by having Black Forest cake smeared all over them?

GOOD SUBSTANCES FOR MESSY PLAY

- Custard
- Cream
- Chocolate sauce
- Massage oil
- Shaving foam
- Gelatin
- Overripe fruit
- Maple syrup

BAD SUBSTANCES FOR MESSY PLAY

- Gas
- Chilli powder
- Vinegar
- Cod-liver oil
- Cat food

TIGHT SPACES

Being confined in a cage, straitjacket, coffin, or rubber body bag may be every claustrophobic's worst nightmare, but to the fetishist who craves sensory deprivation, immobilization, and surrender, it can be a liberating experience. This kind of fetish often goes hand in hand with a love of leather or rubber; these materials feature heavily in confinement scenarios, from whole-body rubber catsuits to leather straitjackets.

MUMMIFICATION

This is the complete immobilization of the body by tightly wrapping it in bandages, bondage tape, plastic wrap, or lycra. Since the head is usually included in the mummification process, it's a means of achieving almost total release from the external world. Fetishists who enjoy this form of restraint may choose to be left for hours in a state of suspended animation, although if you're in charge of someone who is bound this way, it's important never to leave them alone, and always to ensure that airways are free, particularly if the head has been wrapped.

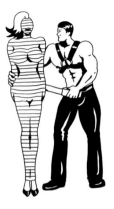

RIGHT, ALL THAT REMAINS IS TO WORK OUT WHERE TO STICK THE STAMPS AND I'LL HAVE YOU IN THE MAIL FIRST THING. . .

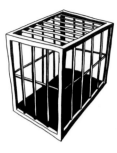

FETISH CAGES ARE OFTEN QUITE SMALL—IDEAL FOR STORING AFTER USE

ZENTAI BODY SUITS

Relatively new on the fetish scene, these are skintight, full head and body suits made of spandex, and available in a full range of different colors. Owing to the nature of spandex, the wearer is able to breathe comfortably through the material and remain encased for long periods of time.

CAGES

While most cages allow a degree of movement, those found in the fetish scene are usually just big enough for a person to stand up or crawl around in. Rather than using a cage for total immobility (though that is easily possible with a few restrainers, rope, or specially made "body" cages), confinement of this variety is usually for games of teasing, chastity, bondage, puppy training, and voyeurism.

SLEEPSACKS

Typically made of rubber or leather, these are body bags that allow the user to be placed inside and zipped up to their neck, leaving the entire body immobile. By placing a collar around the neck or a hood over the head, a greater degree of confinement can also be created. Sleepsacks are designed to permit long-term use; the user may even sleep in them. It must be remembered, however, that encasing the body in materials such as latex and plastic wrap can cause a person to sweat excessively, leading to dehydration; if someone has been kept in this state for a long period of time, it's important that when the session comes to an end they're rehydrated, kept warm, and given a cuddle.

FETISH DICTIONARY

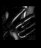

FETİSH

PART FIVE

FETİSH DİCTİONARY

FETISH
DICTIONARY

The fetishizing of particular objects or scenarios is also sometimes referred to as paraphilia. While so far we've dealt primarily with the more common types of fetish practices and behavior, this chapter details a few of the more unusual paraphilias.

As will become clear over the following pages, it is possible to fetishize virtually anything—from the animate to the inanimate, and from teeth to mannequins, even making a lover into a piece of "human furniture."

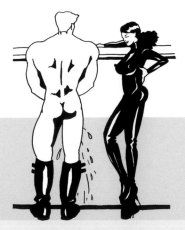

AND A WARM WELCOME
TO UROPHILIACS ANONYMOUS

FETISH DICTIONARY

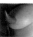

In his day, the composer Wagner was thought by some to be a dangerous subversive because of his fetish for silk and satin. Nowadays these fabrics are considered perfectly acceptable as a means of eroticizing garments. It's worth remembering, therefore, that the fetishes we consider "strange" today may well be the norm tomorrow in a world of ever-evolving sexuality.

ACOMOCLITIC

Hairlessness

An acomoclitic (or smoothie) favors hairlessness, particularly in the genital area. In terms of sexual power play, for a person to be shaved by their partner may be symbolic of a Samson and Delilah relationship. However, whether Delilah lopped off Samson's pubes as well as his head hair, the Bible fails to mention.

AGALMATOPHILISM

Mannequins

An agalmatophile is a person who eroticizes scenarios related to mannequins, robots, or motionless bodies. He or she may, for example, have a strong desire to touch someone who is completely immobilized or unable to prevent themselves from being undressed. Conversely, there may be a desire to be dressed as a mannequin and rendered helpless.

Agalmatophilism is said to exist most frequently among window dressers, who are prone to fantasize about the mannequins they're dressing. Some artists' models, too—after long posing sessions—have admitted to fantasizing about becoming the sculptures themselves, surrendering to the artists' hands, and relishing the sensuous feeling of touch.

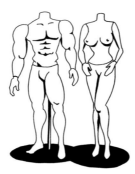

NOT MUCH TO LOOK AT—UNLESS YOU'RE AN AGALMATOPHILE

CAPNOLAGNIA

Smoking

The fetishizing of smoking is believed to be almost exclusive to men. The extent of its popularity has only been fully realized in the past couple of decades, when the rise of the Internet showed a huge demand for images of women, cigarettes dangling carelessly from their lips, staring at the camera.

As a fetish, smoking can be divided loosely into two categories: "glamour smoking" and "dark-side smoking." Glamour smoking relates to the way cigarettes can give women more sexual allure, whether through the image of the bad girl next door or film noir-style sophistication, as exemplified by actresses such as Lauren Bacall, who could make the lighting and inhaling of a cigarette an act of monumental eroticism.

Dark-side smoking, on the other hand, refers to the way cigarettes are used as props in S&M role-play situations. It can include scenarios such as a dominant (dom/domme) or master blowing smoke in a slave's face, using their mouth as an ashtray, making them swallow ash, or even stubbing out cigarettes on their flesh.

Remember: never *mess with the boss. . .*

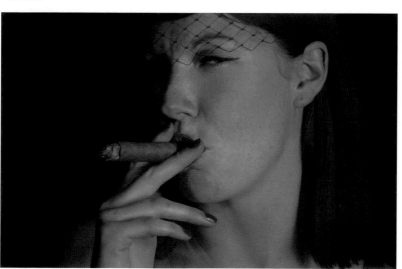

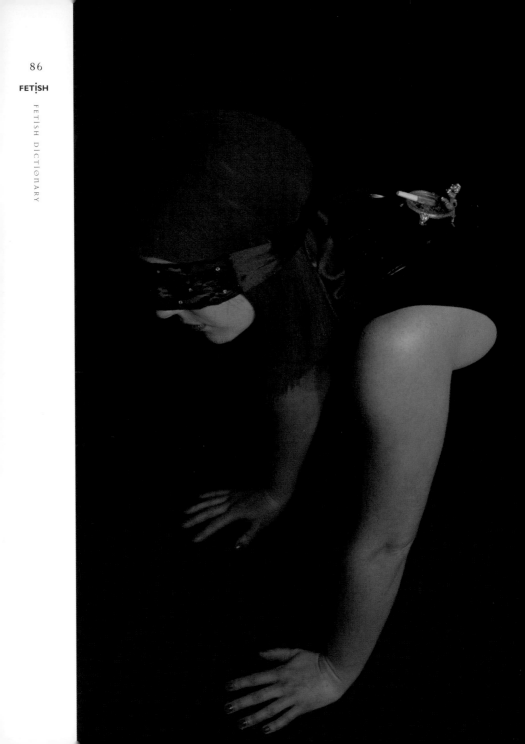

COITUS INTERFERMORIS
Rubbing

Better known as frottaging, dry humping, or scrumping, this involves non-penetrative sexual gratification through the rubbing of the genital area against those of a partners while one or both are fully clothed. Dry humping does not, however, remain restricted to the penis or vagina; it can involve, for example, the rubbing of a man's penis against the breasts, vulva, armpits, or even the feet. For others it may be a pleasurable form of foreplay, but to true fetishists the act of rubbing their genitals against a partner's clothes or boots may be *the* desired sexual act rather than a build-up or replacement of another.

FORNIPHILIA
Furniture

This is a form of sexual objectification in which the dom/domme turns his or her slave into a piece of "human furniture." Most common are human tables, chairs, hat stands, and lampshades, demonstrating that a slave can have a practical use beyond just fawning at their master's or mistress's feet.

To turn a slave into a fashionable coffee table, for example, does require some serious bondage. Forniphilia usually requires complete immobility. For some, this form of play can go on for many hours at a time, with the slave required to remain motionless in the corner covered in hats, or under the weight of his or her owner's legs as they put their feet up and doze off. As a consequence, forniphilia can be potentially hazardous to knee joints and muscles. It's therefore only recommended for those experienced in bondage and aware of a slave's physical limitations.

◄ *Remember never to leave a hot coffee cup on a new table slave; it could leave an unsightly ring*

INFANTILISM

Baby Talk

This is the desire by some adults to wear diapers and be treated as babies. All manner of objects and behavior patterns associated with very early stages of childhood can be incorporated into this fetish, from pacifiers, toys, and baby clothes to wailing, screaming, thumb-sucking, and the inevitable diaper-soiling. Infantilism doesn't, however, equate with a sexual preference for children, as is often assumed because of the sexualization of infant-related paraphernalia. More likely an adult baby will either want to explore their newfound freedom through play, followed by a peaceful doze in their extra-large crib. Or they may wish to succumb to the sexual advances of the dom/domme, usually playing a parent, babysitter, or nanny.

KLISMAPHILIA

Enemas

Usually part of a more complex submissive–dominant role-play (particularly medical scenarios), klismaphilia is the fetish for receiving and giving enemas. It usually involves the naughty sub getting the rubber-tube treatment and having to hold their waters while their sadistic owner looks on and occasionally gives them a spanking for good measure.

Though some couples like to use alcohol in this scenario, it's worth noting that alcohol is absorbed much more quickly by the colon than the stomach, but the colon doesn't have an equivalent vomit reflex if quantities are too extreme. For this reason, if alcohol is being is being used it's essential to dilute it heavily with water to reduce the degree of intoxication of its recipient. And finally, doms/dommes be warned, if you've ever read Stephen King's book *Carrie*, or seen the film, you'll know what happens when you push someone too far...

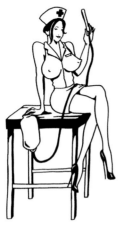

KLISMAPHILIA PUTS A WHOLE NEW SPIN ON THE PHRASE, "THE NURSE IS READY TO SEE YOU NOW, MR SMITH."

LACTOPHILE

Milk

This is a person who is sexually aroused from breast-feeding, or simply being around a lactating woman. We probably don't need Sigmund Freud to explain this one, but if it's not a paraphilia you were aware of previously, it may make you want to reconsider your attitude to breast-feeding in public.

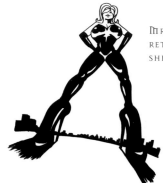

Mrs Gulliver returns—and she's not happy

MACROPHILIA

Big People

A fetish for larger people, macrophilia is usually practiced as part of a bigger game of dominance and submission. Trampling, which involves the sub being used as a human carpet, is a fetish often tied in with giantism: fantasies of towering dommes or doms wandering through the cityscape, crushing slaves beneath their feet like a careless Gulliver. While these kinds of fetishes will hopefully remain merely fantasy, in our lifetime at least, extreme care must still be taken when trampling in high heels across a sub's spine.

DORAPHILIA

Fur or Skin

Many paraphilias focus on contact with a specific item or material, and for doraphiliacs the object of desire is animal fur or skin (i.e. leather). A great deal of fetish clothing and accessories are made from these materials, allowing the individual concerned to wrap themselves from head to toe should they so desire. For some the material conveys a sense of power, as they adopt the character of the animal in whose skin they are clad (this is usually subconscious, although some people deliberately adopt the character of the relevant animal). For others the material conveys a sense of safety and nurturing. As well as the feeling of fur or leather on the body, sexual pleasure can also be derived from the smell that such materials give off.

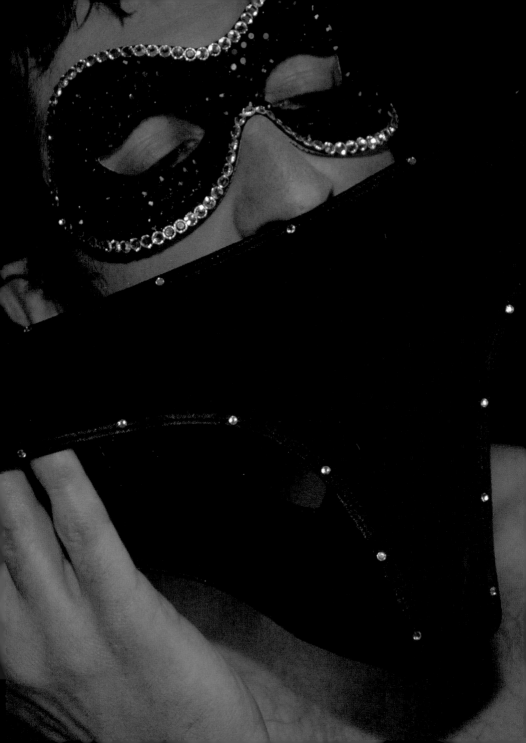

MELCRYPTOVESTIMENTAPHILIA

Black Panties

The sexualizing of silk and satin garments, in many countries, has become so commonplace since the mid-20th century that its appeal is now almost universal. Even the most vanilla of couples will have spiced up their sex life at some point with silky lingerie, hosiery, negligées, a camisole, or even silk boxers. It's the sheen, luster, softness, and elegance of this material that undoubtedly accounts for its popular appeal.

MYSOPHILIA

Used Underwear

Girls' panties have always held an allure for fetishists; often the more soiled the better. Pornographic magazines have been advertising them in their back pages for decades now. While some men like to smell, wear, or fondle the panties, others enjoy masturbating while touching them. Japanese men, for reasons best known to themselves, have a particular fondness for girls dressed as sailors. They'll pay good money for their soiled "bloomers," known as *bura sera* (a loose translation of "Bloomer Sailor"). Dirty panties could even be bought from vending machines around Japan, until complaints were made about it.

◄ *Worn or not worn, that is the question. Soiled panties have long held an allure for fetishists*

ODONTOPHILIA

Teeth

Odontophiliacs are aroused by anything to do with the teeth. As with the shoe fetishist's arousal from getting their tongue around their partner's high heels, many odontophiles like nothing better than licking away the dirt between their partner's molars. Others enjoy having the imprint of their lover's teeth in their skin. Some even get horny from pulling out their partner's teeth. Of course, a mouth only holds so many teeth, so tooth-pulling enthusiasts have to change their lovers often, leaving behind a sorry trail of mumbling mouths.

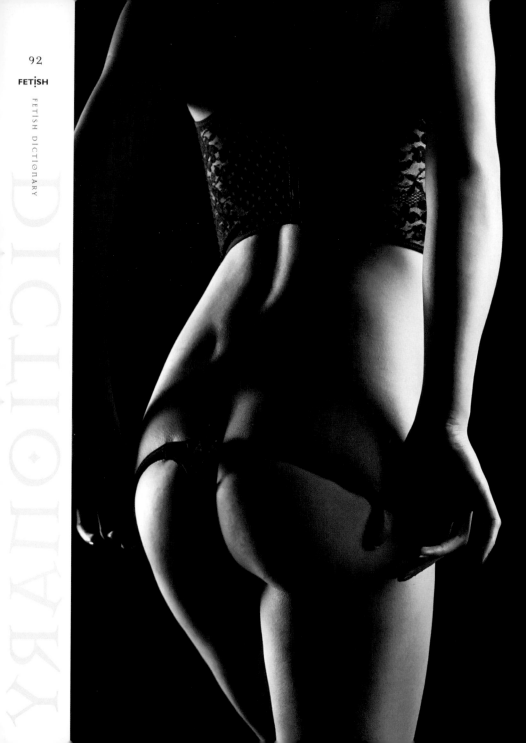

DICTIONARY

*◄ For pygophiliacs, a
lady's rear is worthy of
unadulterated adulation*

PTEROPHILIA
Feathers
Although the use of feathers for tickling a subject's feet is a well-documented turn-on, a specific fetish for feathers is quite rare. The origins of this fetish probably lie in their sensuality, as well as the showy dress outfits and feather boas of stage and screen.

PYGOPHILIA
Ass Worship
Another one almost exclusive to the guys, this is the unadulterated joy of kissing, licking, caressing, and worshiping a lady's bottom. It's also known as "booty worship" and, for the professionals, a "queening stool" can be used. A queening stool is a low seat which fits over the sub's face so he (or she) can't be distracted by the TV or the window cleaner peering in through the patio doors, allowing for uninterrupted adoration of the ass. A word of warning, ass lovers: keep it clean! Fecal bacteria can lead to all sorts of nasty diseases—even STDs.

TRICHOPHILIA
Body Hair
A trichophiliac is aroused by excessive body hair or "hairsuits." This attraction can range from the entire body to specific areas, such as the armpits, anus, or head. According to some advertisements for baldness cures, most women are supposed to be trichophiliacs, although this is, of course, probably a cruel marketing ploy aimed at increasing the insecurity of bald men.

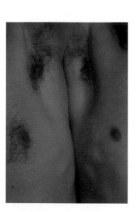

*Body hair—but is this hairy
enough to excite a trichophiliac?*

UROPHILIA
Urine
The sexual attraction to urine (also known as urolagnia) is a common fetish among both men and women. Usually a urophile will be turned on by being urinated on by their partner, although in some cases he or she can also derive pleasure from actually drinking their partner's (or even their own) urine, particularly if in the context of ritualized role-play.

FETISH GEAR

FETİSH GEAR

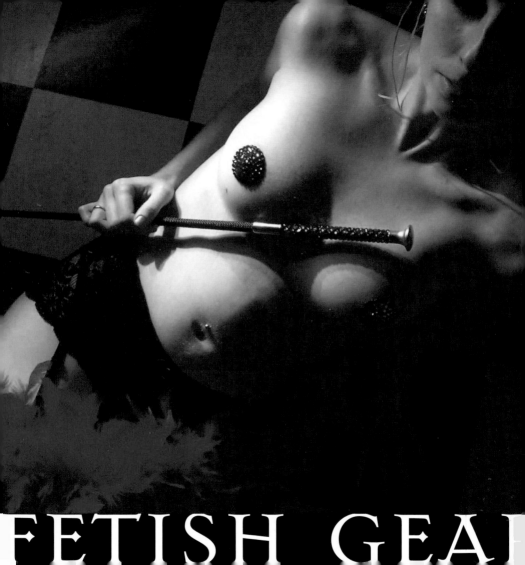

PART SIX

FETISH GEAI

Fetishism or bondage, discipline, sadism, and masochism (BDSM) can be an expensive hobby. There are rubber outfits to be bought, not to mention leather corsets, lingerie, whips, floggers, restraints, collars, chains, cages, canes, and sex toys of every description.

To the ardent fetishist, however, they can offer endless hours of pleasure (and pain). And while this chapter explores a vast range of fetish equipment currently used on the scene, if you really are on the breadline and need whipping into shape, there is a section named Everyday Pervertables (see page 120), listing an array of everyday items that can be used for kinky play.

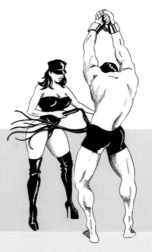

FLOGGING EQUALS BOTH PLEASURE
AND PAIN FOR THE MASOCHIST

RESTRAINTS

A large part of play for many fetishists is bondage. Everything from ropes and chains to bathrobe belts can and has been used over the centuries for sexual power games. While silk scarves remain popular with novices and silk fetishists, ankle and wrist cuffs made of nylon, leather, or metal remain the most common and adaptable forms of restraint.

It's worth bearing in mind, however, that overly complicated buckles, straps, padlocks, or time-consuming knots can turn a kinky session into a laboriously fumbling affair; it's well worth practicing with restraints beforehand to work out how best to apply them with the minimum of fuss and effort.

When using restraints, a safe word must be agreed in case the person tied up begins to find the experience too intense. Phrases like "Stop," "Please don't," or "Ouch, that really hurts, you're a very cruel and sadistic master/mistress," should be avoided, as they can be confusing within the context of the role-playing.

Choose instead a word not usually associated with the situation. It could be anything obvious, from "red" (for stop) to something silly like "rice pudding." If you're using a gag as well as cuffs, then a hand signal should also be agreed. Or a grunt.

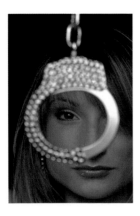

STEEL HANDCUFFS

Originally designed for use by the police in order to temporarily restrain a prisoner, steel handcuffs—while designed for rapid and secure application—can be extremely uncomfortable to wear. If used for kinky play, they must be handled with diligence; misuse or carelessness can cause damage to skin or nerves. It's also worth bearing in mind that under certain circumstances (such as when using steel handcuffs at the same time as lubricants) they can be difficult to remove. And for goodness' sake, make sure you always have a spare key.

BONDAGE TAPE

This specially made shiny, adhesive tape is available from most good fetish stores. It can be applied very quickly and looks good when wrapped around the body parts of a slave (some subs even like to be taken to the fetish club with just a bit of carefully positioned bondage tape around their genitals). Although self-adhesive, one of the major advantages of bondage tape is that it doesn't stick to hair or skin and can be used around the face for gagging without fear of a sub losing their mustache when removed. Disadvantages are mainly its cost—use it liberally and often, and you may have to send your slave out looking for extra work.

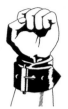

LEATHER HANDCUFFS

Usually attached using buckles (or touch fasteners), the main benefit of leather cuffs over steel ones is that they can be separated and even worn throughout the evening, prior to use. Adjustable and more comfortable than steel handcuffs, some leather cuffs come fur-lined for the ever-demanding sub. However, to ensure there's no chance of his or her escape, they can be padlocked.

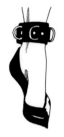

ANKLE CUFFS

While similar in style to leather handcuffs, ankle-restrainers are usually much larger. By using a chain to connect the two cuffs, the dom/domme can restrict the sub's ability to stretch their legs, preventing them from running away.

PLASTIC WRAP

Plastic wrap makes a perfectly good substitute for bondage tape or rope, and can very quickly render the sub immobile. One advantage of plastic wrap is that it can be used effectively for mummification, although care must be taken to ensure it doesn't hamper breathing. Industrial versions of plastic wrap also come in different colors and are made of a heavier-gauge plastic.

LEG SPREADERS

The leg spreader is attached to a pair of ankle restrainers in a similar way to a chain. This simple, straight pole, once secured to the ankles of the sub, keeps the legs forced apart.

Whips, Paddles, and Canes

PADDLES

Usually made of wood or leather, the paddle is a short, portable device for over-the-knee fun and spanking. The best-quality paddles are usually made of maple or ash; the plastic variety are of such inferior quality they're best avoided altogether.

Paddles are safe to use in the hands of even the clumsiest novice, and usually leave the buttocks mark-free, unless in the hands of an over-zealous dom/domme, in which case bruising may appear. For added bite, use a paddle with bevelled holes; this increases the sting by allowing air to pass through, although it can also cause the recipient to bruise more quickly.

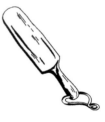

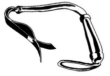

RIDING CROP

A long, flexible handle and one or two short whipping strands make the riding crop a formidable flogger in the right hands. Crops are made of fiberglass rods or canes bound in leather, and were originally used in horseback riding—although servants, grooms, children, and even husbands/wives may well have received a lashing for bad behavior from the master/mistress of the house back in the good old days.

The symbol of a riding crop in BDSM is a strong one: it reminds the slave that they're little more than an animal in their owner's hands.

Riding crops are best used on the back, buttocks, and legs; for those who want something to show for their suffering, crops leave satisfying red stripes on the flesh.

CAT-O'-NINE-TAILS/FLOGGER

Specially developed by the British Navy to keep its naughty
sailors under control, the "cat," rather than having one
long flogger, like most other whips, has many short ones
(traditionally nine). Because the strands are short, floggers are
much easier to control than whips. They also strike a wider
area and are less prone to leaving red stripes on the skin.
Mini-floggers can even be purchased for male and female
genitorture (gentle whipping of the genitals).

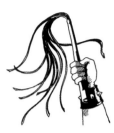

When buying a flogger, check that the tails are all of equal
length, the braiding of the knots tight, and the ends secure.
And give it a swing. The tails of a good flogger should all clump
together; a badly made flogger's tails splay out in all directions.

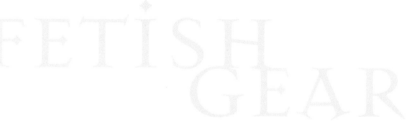

BULLWHIP (OR SINGLE-TAIL WHIP)

The undisputed king of the whips. Bullwhips are highly versatile
and make a satisfying crack, which in itself can be a turn-on
for the user and recipient. They vary according to the rigidity
of their handle and the length of the body or thong. (Shorter
bullwhips are much easier to control in confined spaces.) Any
bullwhip does, however, demand that the user knows what he
or she is doing; there is every chance that some serious harm
can be unwittingly inflicted in the wrong hands. Never crack a
bullwhip toward anyone's face, and always make sure the eyes
are protected when practicing yourself.

TIPS

- When a whip or cane is being
  used, always make sure you have
  a pre-arranged "stop" signal
- Always buy good-quality whips
  and floggers—they'll last longer
  and be safer to use

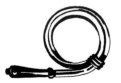

GAGS AND BLINDFOLDS

BALL GAGS

The perfect way to silence a sub. Ball gags may be buckled or strapped to the head and comprise a harness and a leather, rubber, plastic, or foam ball, which—once stuffed into the mouth—parts the teeth and presses the tongue down. Once in place, the wearer can only really communicate through grunts and whines, which of course is half the fun. Ball gags can, however, instigate an unfortunate case of drooling.

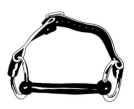

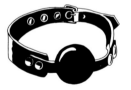

BIT/MUZZLE GAG

The bit gag is similar to a bit for a horse, and is often used in pony play; the muzzle gag is popular for puppy training. Both gags restrict the movement of the jaw, and both come with a head harness. They can have a strong effect on subs and doms/dommes who like the association with the restraining and control of animals.

LAUNDRY

It's important for fetish play to involve at least some degree of improvisation rather than always sticking to the script. For this reason, articles of clothing such as stockings, gloves, and bathrobe belts make great improvised gags. In fact, most male slaves will be thrilled to have their mistress roll up a used stocking into a ball and stuff it into their mouth.

BLINDFOLD

Taking away someone's sight can cause other senses to be magnified dramatically, not to mention the excitement caused by not being able to see what is going to happen next in erotic play. Purpose-made touch-fastening or elasticized blindfolds are best to use in the long run, as makeshift and improvised blindfolds often tend to slip off.

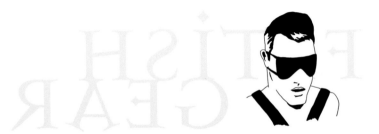

Masks, Collars, and Leashes

LATEX MASKS

A full latex mask—shiny, severe, and stretched tightly over the head—gives total anonymity to the wearer. By removing all facial expressions a mask is a powerful way of de-humanizing the wearer—perfect for those who want to get lost in animal play or add a sense of menace to the one in control. Equally, it can restrict a slave to the point where even their breathing has to be controlled by their owner. Care must be taken that a slave wearing a latex mask can breathe easily, particularly if gagged.

COLLAR AND LEASH

No fetish wardrobe would be complete without a good collar and leash. A leash can be anything from thick chain to a length of rope; collars range from stiff high-neck leather types that restrict movement of the head to a "normal" studded dog collar purchased from a pet store.

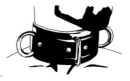

For those who enjoy collar and leash play, a collar with rings allows for the easy removal or attachment of a chain, and also means that a slave can be easily tethered—to a chair leg, bed post, or lamppost, for example.

The physical act of collaring a slave can serve as an ideal start to the ritual of fetish play. Equally, the removal of the collar can signify that play has ended.

It's important to remember that excessive pulling on a collar from behind can damage the throat.

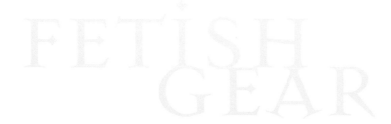

FETISH GEAR

Sex Toys

DILDOS AND VIBRATORS

Dildos are non-vibrating, penis-shaped sex toys that have traditionally been made of rubber, PVC, or chrome. More recently silicon and Pyrex have been employed to create superior-quality dildos and, although more expensive, are recommended as being cleaner and longer-lasting. They may offer a more luxurious sensation, and can be sterilized in boiling water. An added advantage of Pyrex dildos is that they can also be heated to body temperature, or even chilled!

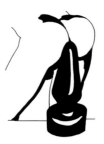

A vibrator is, quite simply, a woman's best friend. Originally, vibrators were invented to cure "female hysteria" in the 1880s, and, incredible though it seems, weren't considered to have anything to do with sexual pleasure. Even more incredible is the fact that they're still deemed illegal in US states such as Texas, and can only be sold if the customer signs a written agreement that the vibrator will only be used for "educational pursuits."

Dildos and vibrators are used extensively in all manner of sex games and play, and while they can be employed for vaginal, clitoral, and anal stimulation, if one is used on the anus it's important to ensure it has a flanged base; if it gets inserted too far it could result in an embarrassing trip to the doctor's.

BUTT PLUGS

These are dildos designed for insertion into the anus. Butt plugs can vary from finger-size to eye-watering dimensions and are usually designed with a flared end to enable them to remain inside the anus, where they can be left for relatively long periods of time. Some subs may be required by their owner to wear a butt plug in public as a reminder of their role (and for discreet pleasure).

To insert a butt plug, large quantities of lubrication and a slow, gentle touch are necessary. Butt plugs should never be shared, and should always be sterilized immediately after use.

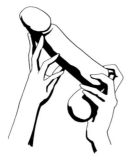

THINK TWICE BEFORE BUYING A NOVELTY-SHAPED DILDO FOR A PARTNER. CHANCES ARE, THEY'D STILL PREFER A CLASSIC PENIS-SHAPE LIKE THIS ONE OVER A CARTOON CHARACTER OR THE EIFFEL TOWER

Nipple Clamps and Clothespins

NIPPLE CLAMPS

Another must-have for most fetishists, nipple clamps can bring a heightened sensitivity to the nipples—a delicious mingling of pain and pleasure. They can also provide a feeling of helplessness, especially if the wearer is tied up and at the mercy of their owner, who may take great delight in gently pulling on the chain that connects the nipples.

Nipple clamps usually come in the form of two alligator clips connected by a chain, although there are plenty of adjustable varieties, allowing the person in charge to keep adding pressure like a thumbscrew. If an even greater degree of pressure is desired, weights may be hung from the clamps. This has the added advantage that if the wearer is being whipped or pleasured in some way, any movement of the body will induce a swinging motion, adding to the gravitational pull on the nipples.

Men (and women to a lesser degree) who claim to have little or no sensitivity in their nipples may find them becoming sensitized through the use of nipple clamps, although a gradual introduction is recommended.

Always make certain that nipple clamps come with a soft plastic or cork ending in order to ensure the nipples are safeguarded from unnecessary chafing or tearing.

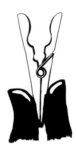

CLOTHESPINS

Though not the most aesthetically pleasing fetish accessory, clothespins can be found in most households and offer a versatility not provided by nipple clamps. While they can't be adjusted like most clamps, pins *can* be attached to most parts of the flesh, not just nipples but genitals, breasts, earlobes, lips, and tongue. Those with a higher pain threshold often enjoy a line of pins on particular areas of the flesh, which are linked with a length of string and whipped off like a zipper. Ouch!

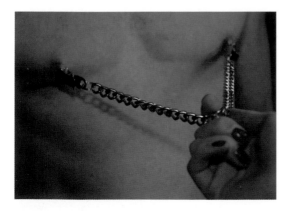

FETISH GEAR

STRAP-ONS

These are dildos or vibrators attached to a harness that is worn around the user's lower abdomen or thigh and serve as an alternative to a penis for intercourse.

A strap-on, if used properly, is going to take a good battering, and as with most sex toys, quality pays in the long run. As with standard dildos and vibrators, it's best to go for a durable but flexible material such as silicon. As for size and shape, that's purely down to taste. If you're introducing your (male) partner to strap-on sex for the first time, it may be wise to go for something smaller or thinner than a standard penis-sized dildo, to break him in gently. You don't want to scare him off by wandering into the bedroom with "the Beast" between your legs for the first time. And, once he's gotten used to a smaller strap-on, you can upgrade at a later date.

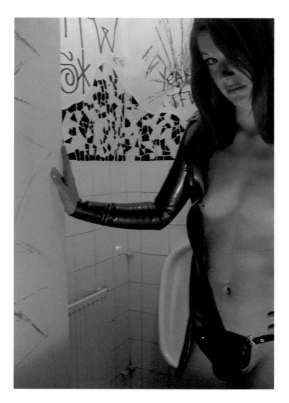

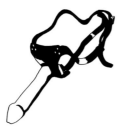

Some strap-ons are glued into garments such as rubber underwear or bodices, although more often they come as two separate items: dildo and harness. Both are important. If a harness is flimsy or only has two straps to go around the waist, it may not be enough to hold the dildo firmly in place, leading to chafing.

Three or four straps are preferable—the extra ones can be tied around the thighs or under the groin, giving greater support.

As with all sex toys designed for penetration, good lubrication and sterilization are essential.

Cages and Straitjackets

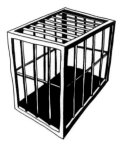

CAGES

When a slave has been especially naughty, what do you do with them? You lock them in their cage, of course. And for those who enjoy playing roles of animal and trainer, voyeur and exhibitionist, teased and chastised, master and servant, etc., the cage is the ultimate accessory for demonstrating who's boss. The most popular cage design in the fetish market is currently the "puppy"—a steel-tubed box with enough space for a naughty slave/dog to crawl into and either squat, curl up, or kneel.

Because of the bars, the slave can be totally restrained inside in any number of ways and for as long as necessary, while you invite the neighbors over for dinner and leave him or her in the corner to be fed tidbits, if well-behaved. The design of the puppy cage is such that it can be dismantled easily—useful to know, should parents suddenly choose to make a surprise visit.

STRAITJACKETS

Though traditionally used for restraining patients in hospital who may cause harm to themselves or others, in the fetish world the straitjacket is a perfect means of rendering a slave immobile around the torso. The arms of a straitjacket are sewn at the ends, folded over the front of the body, and strapped together at the back—ideal for the sub who can't stop fidgeting with their hands.

Despite the common scene of an escapologist struggling free from the shackles of a straitjacket, the only way a person can liberate themselves from a proper straitjacket is by having the ability to dislocate the shoulders, something the great magician Houdini was apparently capable of doing. (For the less dextrous escapologist, an oversized or gimmicked jacket is usually the secret to their liberation.)

Because of the relative expense of a straitjacket (particularly high-quality custom-made leather ones), they're rarely found in the fetish novice's wardrobe.

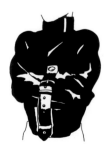

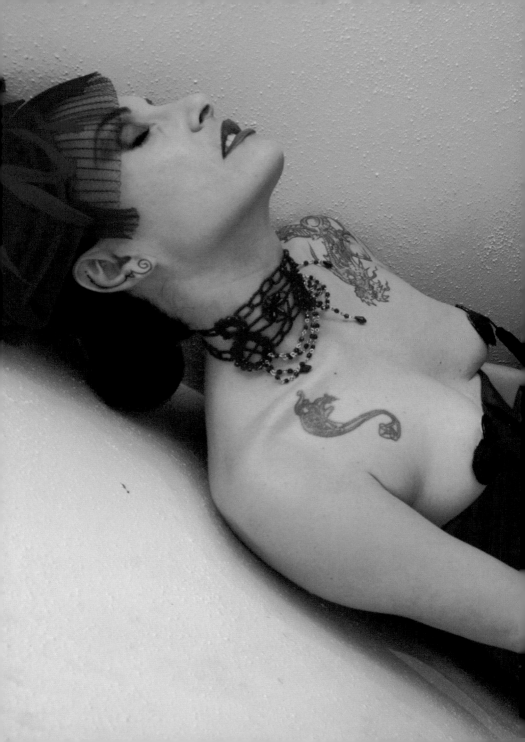

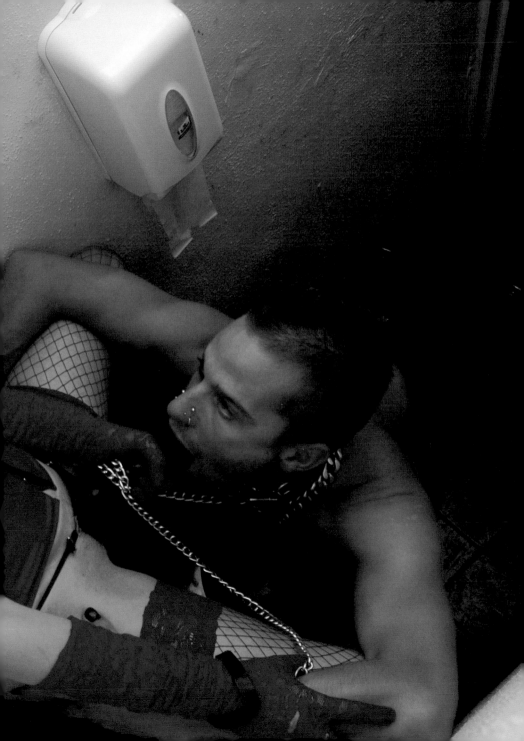

Violet Wands

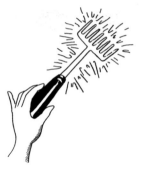

Violet Wands have actually been around since the 1930s, when they were first sold as skin and muscle toners and hair restorers! They simply plug into the wall and—when placed near the body—create an electricity transfer (in the form of a burst of small blue sparks) accompanied by a satisfying buzz and the feeling of "being walked on by a kitten with its claws out." The thrill induced is, in fact, an adrenalin and endorphin rush brought on by the shock. Wands can be applied anywhere on the body but should be kept away from the head, eyes, and *all* orifices: they're made of thin glass and can easily break. It's also best not to use a violet wand on someone with a heart condition or pacemaker, unless you're after their inheritance.

Cock Rings

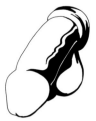

A cock ring is a circular piece of material worn around the base of the penis and testicles, often to help the wearer maintain an erection but sometimes simply for the pleasing pressure it exerts on the genital area. Hard cock rings made of metal or plastic need to be slipped over the penis and testicles before erection takes place, and usually cannot be removed until the penis is soft again, a fact which, in itself, can add a sense of extra excitement.

Other varieties can be made of elastic or stretch Velcro, which allow the wearer to adjust the tightness of the cock ring and slip it on and off at their leisure.

It does, however, need to be mentioned that wearing a tight metal cock ring for too long can cause damage to the penis; if left on indefinitely it can eventually lead to the penis dropping off, and nobody wants that.

CHASTITY BELTS

These are locking devices that can be fitted around a man's or woman's genital region to prevent the wearer from engaging in sexual intercourse or masturbation. For women the chastity device usually takes the form of a plastic or metal belt which fits around the pelvis like a thong. For men it comprises a plastic or metal locking cage that fits around the testicles and penis, preventing erections. Used in long-term psychological sex games, a chastity belt can be worn for several weeks without any harm, and is often used for role-play involving teasing and denial.

For men the belt can be a particularly tough challenge: the wearer must train his mind not to focus on the erotic nature of the game, otherwise this will lead to sexual arousal, an erection, and extreme discomfort. It can be a vicious circle, but then that's part of the training and the fun.

For those keen to indulge in long-term play with chastity belts, it's best to buy plastic not metal ones if traveling by plane; passing through customs could get a trifle embarrassing. . .

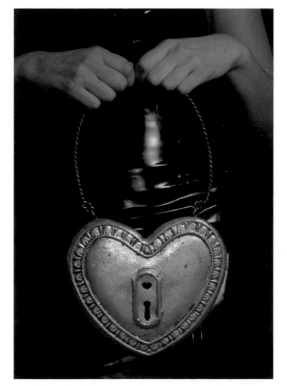

Clothing

Fetish dress can cover a whole spectrum of clothing, from a full rubber nurse's uniform to soiled panties. It's often the strong identification a person has with the clothing that forms the fetish; in other cases it's the material itself. It can't be denied, however, that tight, shiny, figure-hugging materials such as rubber, leather, and PVC dominate the fetish world and still account for the majority of the clothing worn on the scene.

There is something exciting, taboo, and provocative about a woman in a tight rubber dress or a man in shiny leather. A seemingly innocent PVC raincoat on the street will turn many heads, as will a leather skirt. There is something alluring about the way these materials cling to the body and shine and ripple over the body's contours as it moves. For some people it's the thrill of restriction brought on from wearing such clothes (a tight skirt, for example); for others it's the smell (leather pants), the sound they make (the rustle of PVC on stockinged legs, the creak of leather), or the way the material glides with the body (rubber dress).

Even most non-fetishists will admit to the allure of seeing their partner in something tight, black, shiny, and slinky. Almost every conceivable item of clothing can be purchased now in rubber, leather, or PVC, although many fetishists still have their clothes specially made, to cater for specific kinks and desires. There are, however, enduring kinky favorites, a few of which are listed here.

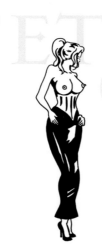

THE HOBBLE SKIRT

A fetish classic, the hobble is an ankle-length skirt that hugs the legs all the way down to the feet, restricting the wearer's ability to walk (turning it almost into a shuffle). The hobble first came into fashion in the 1880s, although today's kinky designs are closer in style to those worn in the 1910s. For those who love to feel restricted in fetish clothing, the hobble skirt and corset make a perfect combination.

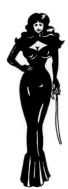

THE MISTRESS DRESS

As is often the case with fetish, it's a question of how much of the body you can't see or access—not how much you can—hence the allure of the mistress dress. With its high neck, long sleeves, and skirt reaching either to the knees or down to the ankles, this design restricts access to most parts of the body and is worn to tease and control, or to be teased and controlled in.

FRENCH MAID

No fetish uniform has quite enjoyed the mass erotic appeal as the French maid outfit. Whether made with satin, cotton, rubber, leather, or PVC, it remains a perennial favorite, from couples wanting to bring a little sauciness into their sex life to cross-dressing servile men. It's amazing what a bit of lace and an apron can do for the libido.

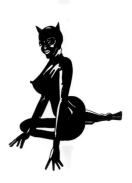

CATSUIT

The classic second skin, the catsuit first appeared in the 1940s (when it was actually knitted!) and was popularized through the cult TV show *The Avengers*. Nowadays rubber, PVC, and leather are the preferred materials for showing off the contours of the body with a catsuit. No fetish wardrobe should be without one!

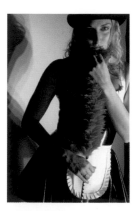

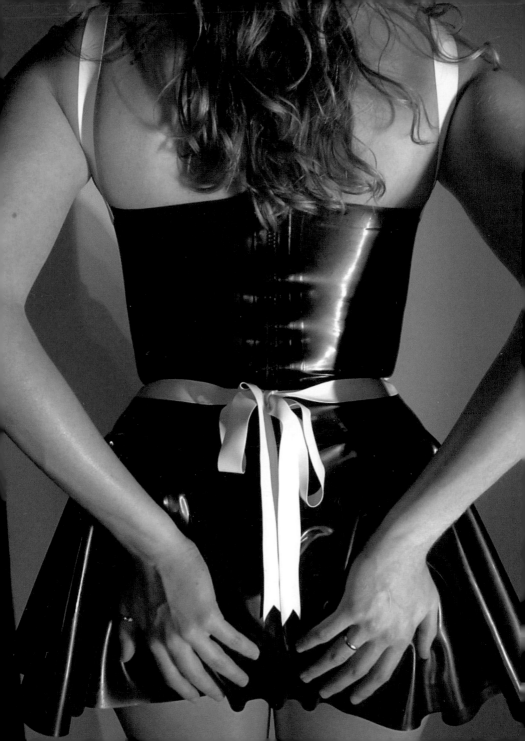

FETISH MATERIALS

PVC

PVC is a friendly fetish material. It's not a struggle to put on, it allows the skin a chance to breathe, and it's usually cheaper than rubber and leather. It also doesn't expose every bump and blob of cellulite, making it a little kinder on the eye for those who don't have the body of a supermodel. The downside is that over time PVC tends to bubble and blister. To many on the fetish scene, PVC is the poor cousin to rubber.

There are a lot of cheap and badly made PVC garments on the market, and it pays to buy from a reputable manufacturer. Unlike rubber and leather, however, alterations are easy and relatively inexpensive.

Real PVC is rarely used these days in fetish clothing; it doesn't stretch, and cracks easily. PU (polyurethane) is used instead.

PVC CARE

- *PVC should be hand-washed (to last longer) in warm water, and hung to dry inside out.*
- *It can be polished with a silicon spray.*

LEATHER

Leather is a relatively common fetish; although it's often associated with the BDSM side of the gay community, who's going to deny that Jim Morrison pouting in his leather pants, or Lucy Liu's office bitch in a leather suit, cracking the whip in *Charlie's Angels*, did look spectacularly sexy in leather?

Even more than with rubber and PVC, it pays to try on leather before you buy it, because of its cost. Being stiff, however, it doesn't cling to the body's contours quite as severely as rubber.

LEATHER CARE

- *Wipe with a damp cloth to remove stains*
- *Regularly use a good-quality leather polish to keep it in good condition*

RUBBER/LATEX

Unlike leather and PVC, rubber is almost exclusively associated with fetish. The wearing of rubber is a labor of love. It shows every lump of the body, and it can also be hard to put on—often requiring copious amounts of talcum powder or lube. It can make the wearer uncomfortably sweaty and, once ripped, it's extremely difficult to repair. But if you're a rubber fetishist you'll also appreciate that nothing on earth feels like it, smells like it, or looks so good.

When buying rubber it always pays to go for high-quality brands; the rubber garments will be more durable, better made, and will usually polish up with a better sheen.

RUBBER CARE

- *To clean rubber, wear it in the shower and wash with a non-greasy soap-based lubricant, both inside and out, then hang it up to dry (away from a radiator!)*
- *Always hang rubber up rather than folding it away in drawers*
- *Avoid contact with oil-based lubricants and creams when wearing latex*

Lingerie

Even the most vanilla of couples are likely to have a bit of racy underwear somewhere in the closet, whether it's lacy panties, silk camisoles, baby-doll nighties, stockings and garter belts, fishnets, or the odd satin slip. In the fetish world, all this is embraced, and more besides. While most non-cross-dressing men have to make do with rubber briefs, silk boxers, and g-strings, an embarrassment of riches is available for the ladies.

Complete outfits of stockings, garter belts, and bras in rubber, leather, PVC, satin, and lace of every possible design, shape, and color are available. These can be combined with dog collars, gloves, hoods, boots, high heels, or even used as nighttime clubwear. Fetish lingerie can also be worn in secret underneath everyday clothes to thrill an unsuspecting partner at the appropriate (or not so appropriate) time.

Countless men, of course, also get a thrill from wearing women's lingerie themselves, and finding a partner sympathetic to this fetish can be a great source of comfort. If a male partner has a fetish for underwear, the kindest thing you can do is indulge their pleasure and buy them their dream attire; for a fetishist there is no greater joy.

I WAS GOING TO MAKE A JOKE ABOUT A "FREUDIAN SLIP," BUT THEN THOUGHT BETTER OF IT

TIPS FOR BUYING FETISH LINGERIE:

- *Would a peephole bra and crotchless panties be better than a standard bra and panties for the kind of games you have planned?*
- *For men buying female underwear, remember to measure your chest, AND padding to get an idea of what size bra you might need. If in doubt about cup size, stick with a B.*

GLOVES

Whether cuff-length black leather, tight latex, satin opera-style, or regular domestic ones in banana yellow, gloves are an essential part of the fetish wardrobe. They add menace to a uniform, elegance to a dress, and kinkiness to a medical game. For glove fetishists there is something sublime about a hand encased in shiny black material holding a dog collar, caressing a cigarette, or clutching a whip.

As with much fetish clothing, the allure of gloves lies in the covering of the body, the mystery of the second skin, the transfer of power to the wearer. A man in a suit won't stand out from the crowd, but when dressed in a pair of black leather gloves there is something creepy, powerful, and mysterious about him.

For those who want an easy life, elbow-length PVC or satin gloves slip on and off with ease compared to latex, and are ideal for those who like to see their partners up to their elbows in black shiny material. But remember, fetish isn't about making things easy; if you prefer rubber, wear rubber.

TIPS FOR BUYING/ WEARING ELBOW-LENGTH RUBBER GLOVES

* *Check that the gloves aren't too baggy around the wrist and upper arm*
* *If you can, try them on: if they're too loose they'll look cheap; if they're too tight they'll cut off your blood circulation and soon begin to hurt*
* *To ensure a rubber glove slips on easily, either fill it with talcum powder or turn the glove inside out and rub it with a non-oil-based lube. (The advantage of the lube is that there won't be talc all over the floor when you take them off.)*
* *Before putting on a long rubber glove, blow it up gently like a balloon until any fingers that may have tucked in from previous wear have popped out*
* *Wrinkle the glove up and put it on carefully, just as you would a stocking*
* *Remove it with similar care*

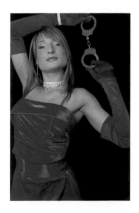

CORSETS

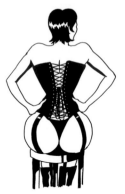

Popularized in the Victorian era, when they were worn almost exclusively by women, corsets were designed to dramatically reduce the wearer's waistline and exaggerate the hips, creating the classic wasp or hourglass figure. Up until relatively recently corsets fell out of fashion, but they have enjoyed a big revival thanks to their growing appeal in the fetish, goth, and burlesque scene. They're now worn as both inner and outer garments, and favored by any man or woman who enjoys the sensation of restriction and modification of the shape of the torso.

Modern corsets are typically made of such malleable materials as leather or cloth, and are stiffened (or "boned") with the addition of plastic or steel strips inserted inside the material, like ribs.

To achieve their tightness, corsets are laced from the back. To do this without help is near-impossible, unless you're a yoga expert with arms the length of a baboon. Traditionally the lacing of a corset would have been the job of a lady-in-waiting. Nowadays, it's the role of the partner, spouse, gimp, slave, or a well-trained pet monkey.

HOW TO TIE A CORSET

Tying a corset may appear daunting to the novice but is, in fact, relatively straightforward and rather like tying a shoelace.

- *Start at the top; it's easier to work down rather than up.*
- *As with a boot, poke each separate lace through the eyelets on left and right at the top of the corset to leave two even lengths of lace.*
- *Thread the lace on the right through the next eyelet on the left.*
- *Thread the lace on the left through the next eyelet on the right.*
- *Continue until you reach the waist in the center of the corset.*

- *Take the lace on the left and loop it into the eyelet below (also on the left).*
- *Take the lace on the right and loop it into the eyelet below (also on the right).*
- *Ensuring the loops remain, continue lacing as before until you reach the bottom of the corset.*
- *Tie the laces into a strong knot.*
- *To adjust the tightness of the corset (and to achieve that wasp-like figure) pull on the excess lengths of the loops.*

Check with the person wearing the corset that it isn't too tight. If they have gone blue, stopped breathing, and are waving their hands in the air like a lunatic, you may need to loosen it a little.

BOOTS AND SHOES

For many people, there is nothing more deliciously sexy that a slim pair of legs in a pair of high heels, but in the fetish world almost anything related to footwear can be— and has been—eroticized. Whether hobbling around the house in a partner's five-inch thigh-high boots, licking the dirt from a black shiny stiletto, sniffing an old sweaty sneaker, cleaning a partner's army boots, or relishing the satisfying sound of the zipper snapping up your leg as you don your favorite knee-high patent leather riding boots, a whole world of fetish exists exclusively for footwear.

For some fetishists, the height of a heel can be more important than the shoe or boot itself. Anything from one to six inches can be hobbled around in without too much fear of falling, although if it's your first time in a pair of killer heels, it's worth practicing your walk before facing the outside world. In fact, when buying a pair of kinky shoes or boots, it's always worth considering the size of the heel in relation to what you'll be wearing them for. If they're purely for bedroom fun, then the sky's the limit. But if you want a pair of heels for towering over your slave as you make them crawl beside you at a club, or just for the pleasure of clicking down the street feeling powerful and sexy, the fantasy of impossibly high heels can quickly become an uncomfortable experience. But as we've already established, fetishism is all about style over comfort— and besides, you can always take it out on your slave when you get home.

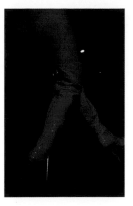

TIPS ON BUYING THIGH-HIGH BOOTS

- *Check how wide the top of the boot is: while some fetishists prefer the "fishing boot" look, a slimmer fit around the thigh is usually considered more elegant.*

- *Ensure the contours of the boot from ankle to thigh follow the leg rather than sag.*

- *It pays to choose boots that zip or lace up, rather than ones that stretch and hold with elastic; these tend to wrinkle quickly and can make the wearer look like a kinky grandma in PVC stockings.*

- *For men buying boots (or stilettos) for the first time, it pays to get specially made footwear from cross-dressing suppliers, as they're usually made with the extra weight in mind, meaning you're less likely to break a heel and fall flat on your face at that all-important dinner party.*

Piercing and Body Jewelry

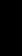 Piercing has always been strongly associated with the fetish scene. It includes many of the classic aspects of fetishism: ritual, pain, body modification, and the objectification and eroticizing of body parts.

While pierced ears have long been socially acceptable, the past couple of decades have seen the rise of the "modern primitive" and a huge increase in tongue, eyebrow, lip, nose, and genital piercings. This ever-evolving scene now includes piercings for the anus, the back of the neck, branding, and the insertion of metal plates beneath the skin. If someone could figure out how to pierce tonsils, no doubt we'd all be sporting those, too.

In fetish role-play, piercings can add spice, elegance, and allure. They can also be used directly for sex games—a sub with pierced nipples or genitals can be led around (very carefully!) on a leash, for example.

Don't. however, always expect that a new piercing is going to make a part of your body suddenly feel more "alive." For some people a piercing can bring heightened sensitivity, but for others it can have the opposite effect.

Using a professional piercer with an impeccable reputation for hygiene cannot be recommended highly enough. Allergic reactions and bacterial and parasitic infections remain relatively common side effects of piercings. Surgical stainless steel and titanium are still considered the safest metals for new piercings, particularly for sensitive areas.

EVERYDAY PERVERTABLES

- *Gags/bits: rubber bones for pets, and golf balls*
- *Collars and leashes: visit the local pet store*
- *Whip handles: bicycle handle grips*
- *Rubber whips: slice an old bicycle inner tube*
- *Paddles: table-tennis bats*
- *Canes: plastic coat hangers*
- *Nipple clamps: clothespins*
- *Floggers: leather belt, hairbrush, wooden spoons, spatulas*
- *Bondage tape: freezer tape*
- *Hot wax play: household candles*
- *Mummification: plastic wrap*
- *Pony play: crops, stirrups, and bits can all be purchased at horseback riding stores*

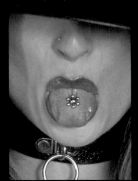

EROTIC PIERCINGS

NIPPLES
This highly sensitive
erogenous zone can be
pierced in both men and
women. Rings remain the
most popular type of jewelry
for this area.

Male Genitals:

AMPALLANG
One of the more popular
piercings for the penis, the
ampallang is a bar that passes
horizontally through the glans.

PRINCE ALBERT
This is a piercing that goes
from the urethra on the glans,
to the outside of the penis.

HAFDA
This term refers to any
piercing that passes through
the scrotum (or ball sack).

Female Genitals:

INNER AND OUTER LABIA
Piercings can be done through
one or both sides of the outer
labia and a ring added near the
opening if desired.

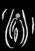

PREPUCE
This piercing goes through
the clitoris hood, and there's
often a tiny ball on the ring
for stimulation.

CLITORAL
Piercing of the clitoris is rare
and not recommended; the
area is small, inaccessible, and
extremely sensitive.

FETISH ARTS

PART SEVEN

FETISH

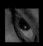

FETİSH

PART SEVEN

FETİSH ARTS

FETISH ARTS

Fetish themes are almost commonplace these days in contemporary culture, be it kinky rubber outfits in Hollywood movies, fetish-themed clothes on the catwalk, Angelina Jolie talking about her perversions in the papers, or the memoirs of a dominatrix becoming a new bestseller.

As everyone knows, sex sells, and fetishism nowadays appears to be the icing on the cake. Whether this is mere fashion, zeitgeist, or proof that fetishism as a way of life is becoming more mainstream remains to be seen.

Good works of art with fetish themes at their core, however, remain few and far between. This chapter highlights the best of what's currently on offer.

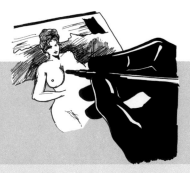

HIGH-QUALITY SPECIALIST FETISH
ART IS A RARE COMMODITY

FETISH IN THE MOVIES

THE IMAGE OR PUNISHMENT OF ANNE

(Dir. Radley Metzger, 1976)
Based on the novel of the same name, this superior art-porn flick centers on the relationship between a trio of Parisian sophisticates: a domme, her harangued slave (Anne), and the film's narrator, Jean. When not being made to have intercourse with store assistants, tied up and whipped in her mistress's dungeon, or having roses stuck where the sun doesn't shine, Anne is handed over to Jean for him to use as he pleases. It doesn't take long before he's fully immersed in the game, and soon everyone's having a good time apart from Anne. Her cold, impassive face does lend a slightly disquieting portrait of her as victim rather than willing participant, particularly since she goes a bit crazy at the end and turns on her mistress. If you can swallow the seventies misogyny, the sex scenes are genuinely erotic and leave little to the imagination. Not an easy film to track down, but fans of the book should find it a real treat and a worthy interpretation.

IN THE REALM OF THE SENSES

(Dir. Nagisa Oshima, 1977)
A graphic tale of sexual obsession in 1930s Japan that leads to a chilling conclusion. Both a celebration of passion and a warning to those who just can't get "enough."

BELLE DE JOUR

(Dir. Luis Buñuel, 1967)
Catherine Deneuve, a bored housewife, takes to prostitution to get her kicks, and spends the rest of her time fantasizing about being dominated. Great outfits; silly story.

MAÎTRESSE/MISTRESS

(Dir. Barbet Schroeder, 1976)
A young Gérard Depardieu plays a thief who gets more than he bargained for when he attempts to burgle the house of a domme. While the film's moralistic tone is deeply irritating (thief converts unhappy domme into nice little housewife), there are some good scenes in the mistress's dungeon, helped by the fact that the slaves, rather than being professional actors, were actually real subs from the Parisian fetish scene.

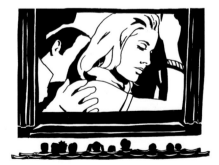

MOVIES

PREACHING TO THE PERVERTED
(Dir. Stuart Urban, 1997)
Trust the British to dream up a fetish political comedy. But then we all know what a bunch of perverts they are behind closed doors. Urban's film follows the exploits of a government minister's sidekick who decides to crack down on S&Mers to show the public his political party has high morals. But he ends up falling for a domme—not that unlikely, given the track record of British politicians. While full of clever, funny, and wry observations about the hypocrisy of those who wield the power, it's worth noting that *Preaching to the Perverted* is a comedy with a fetish theme. Though there are no "heavy" scenes for those wanting some serious S&M titillation, seeing the film's central character, Guinevere Turner, swanning around in hot rubber outfits is a thoroughly satisfying experience.

NIGHT PORTER
(Dir. Liliana Cavani, 1974)
An S&M relationship between a former concentration-camp guard (Dirk Bogarde) and his lover (Charlotte Rampling) is rekindled when Rampling enters a hotel in postwar Germany to find Bogarde working there as a porter. A kinky, disturbing, and very watchable movie.

SECRETARY
(Dir. Steven Shainberg, 2002)
Boss and secretary, James Spader and Maggie Gyllenhaal, turn master and servant in this light-hearted, but very kinky, romantic comedy. There's plenty of spanking, caning, masturbation, and humiliation. Something for the whole family.

ONES TO AVOID:

9 1/2 WEEKS
(Dir. Adrian Lyne, 1986)
A furry handcuffs-style BDSM relationship between Mickey Rourke and Kim Basinger, and a film that takes itself way too seriously for the harmless piece of fluff that it is.

SALO
(Dir. Pier Paolo Pasolini, 1976)
The Marquis de Sade's *120 Days of Sodom* translated to 1940s Italy is more a meditation on the horror of fascism than a kinky romp through sadomasochism. Overblown, too long, and with a rather stomach-churning shit-eating scene that may make you feel too sick to eat for days.

THE STORY OF "O"
(Dir. Just Jaeckin, 1975)
Don't be drawn in by the title—this film is like a pizza with the base and tomatoes taken away: all cheese.

VENUS IN FURS
Several films have been made in the past forty years based on Sacher-Masoch's book—each as dull as the rest.

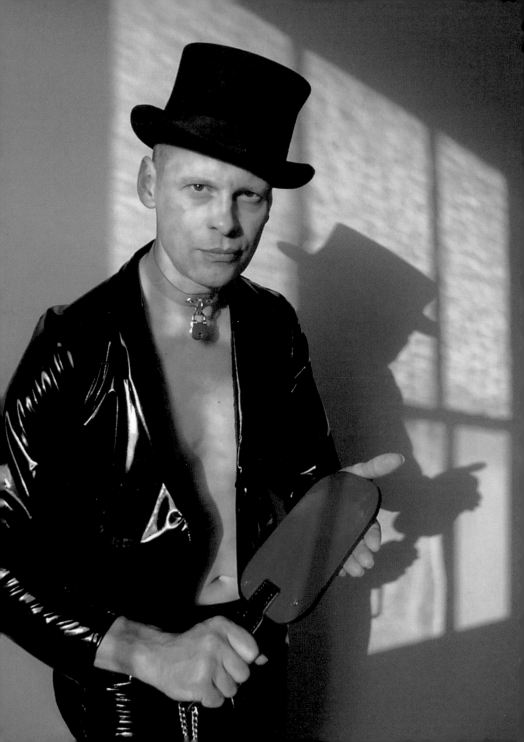

FETISH DOCUMENTARIES

FETISHES

(Dir. Nick Broomfield, 1996)
Gonzo documentary
filmmaker Nick Broomfield
opens the doors on one of
New York's most famous
and exclusive S&M parlors—
Pandora's Box—run by the
enigmatic and mischievous
Mistress Raven. As a fly-on-
the-wall documentary the
film is spot-on, giving a rich
insight into the lives of the
girls who work there and
their clients. It also manages
to explore a wide range
of different fetishes, from
wrestling to infantilism to
rubber. Broomfield keeps his
editing as raw as ever, and
there are some genuinely
uncomfortable moments. For
example, one client turns
aggressive during a wrestling
match and has to be ejected,
and in one incident Nick
oversteps the boundaries
and gets yelled at by the girls.
But, while Broomfield's voice
remains impartial throughout
the film, his unwillingness to
sample one of their "sessions"
clearly frustrates some of the
mistresses. One of the film's
highlights finds Broomfield
pilloried and squirming in a
corner while the girls attempt
to tie him up and whip him.
Unfortunately he escapes.

SICK: THE LIFE AND DEATH OF BOB FLANAGAN, SUPERMASOCHIST

(Dir. Kirby Dick, 1997)
It all begins with Bob
cheerfully writing his obituary.
He is dying from Cystic
Fibrosis (CF) and this film is
a documentary of the last
few years of his life. While
most CF suffers die by their
early twenties, Bob made it
to his early forties, a fact he
attributed to his "healthy" sex
life. And what a sex life it was!

One of the really touching
aspects of *Sick* is the loving
relationship between Bob
and his girlfriend, Sheree, who
acted not only as a soulmate
and domme, but also as a
full-time carer when Bob's
condition became unbearable.

If you're squeamish about
body parts being mutilated
with blunt instruments, you
may want to leave the room
when Bob starts singing
Hammer of Love. Otherwise,
this compelling and touching
documentary is thoroughly
recommended, not least for
demonstrating that deep,
loving relationships and
extreme S&M play aren't
mutually exclusive.

BEYOND VANILLA

(Dir. Claes Lilja, 2001)
Gone are the days when
fetish documentaries used
to be presented by some
humorless ex-MTV presenter
dressed in a tattered rubber
dress, droning on about "the
scene," with bored-looking
actors in a badly lit studio
pretending to whip each
other with sticks of celery.
In this documentary, Lilja has
really done a first-class job.
He covers a broad spectrum
of fetishes through vox-
pops and interviews, with
everyone from porn stars
to housewives. Real-life S&M
scenarios are also filmed,
many of which really do go
"beyond vanilla." There are
demonstrations with different
equipment and toys, tips
of what to do and what to
avoid, and even paternal
advice from the director
about the importance of
trust and commitment.

CLASSIC FETISH PORN

THE FASHIONISTAS
(Dir. John Stagliano, 2002)
Since its release, *Fashionistas* has set a new standard for adult movies that remains unsurpassed. It went on to win just about every accolade and award going in the industry, and deservedly so. It looks like a high-budget motion picture, is over four hours long, shot on 35mm film, professionally lit, and incorporates an extensive and lavish array of rubber and PVC costumes. The only thing that's missing is long, funky wah-wah guitar solos during the orgies.

As with all good porn films, the plot, while probably well-scripted (for porn standards), is utterly dispensable, and the acting passable at best. But let's face it—these things only get in the way.

The Fashionistas' slick and varied platter of pornography ranges from face-slapping, whipping, and group gangbangs to some pretty hardcore scenes, which may be a little extreme for the S&M novice. If it does hit the mark and leave you hungry for more, however, there's even a sequel.

GWEN MEDIA
This LA-based film company has been knocking out fetish movies for years now and has earned a deserved reputation for delivering short, but high-quality, softcore, glossy S&M films. Virtually all of Gwen Media's movies are girl-on-girl action, and while scenarios, themes, and costumes vary wildly, you can generally expect a bit of light domination, discipline, encasement, hot wax, whipping, and the like. Where Gwen Media score highly is for those who want to see attractive girls in rubber tottering around in heels and being dominant.

Its catalog is far too extensive for individual recommendations; best to scroll through the reviews on its website and take your pick.

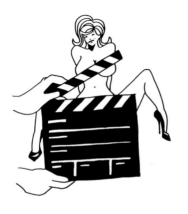

ERIC STANTON

A pioneer in fetish illustration and comic-book art, Stanton began creating kinky cartoons in the 1950s and continued up until his death in the late 1990s. His strips focus largely on the theme of female domination, with feisty wives and girlfriends taking revenge on their lovers for (real or imagined) misdemeanors, resulting in bondage and beatings. Stanton's artwork is detailed, colorful, often humorous, and genuinely erotic. As with other artists working in the fetish field in the 1950s and 1960s, many of his illustrations were actually drawn to order. Nowadays, Stanton's catalog of work can be found in coffee-table-style glossy books which are well worth poring over, particularly if you've got a slave who's willing to be your coffee table.

SARDAX

This highly original and unusual fetish artist has been working with watercolors and Indian ink for over twenty years to create his very own surreal fantasyland (Sartopia), an amorphous landscape that changes from tropical rainforest to Victorian England. His works feature oriental prison guards, regal women in fur, and even Egyptian goddesses riding giant scarab beetles. In Sartopia, Sardax's whip-wielding goddesses rule supreme over scantily clad and tormented men, who are often in the throes of agony and ecstasy as they pull on dog-sleds or are led around on all fours.

DORIS KLOSTER

A world-renowned photographer and filmmaker, Kloster specializes in using realistic settings for her work, as apposed to "artificial" studio scenarios. Her photographs are taken in dungeons and real-life locations all around the world and feature professional dommes and their slaves. Fans of The Story of "O" might be interested to know that Kloster turned this into a beautiful and lavish full-length photo story, together with original text from the novel.

FETiSH FiCTiON

VENUS iN FURS

(Leopold von Sacher-Masoch)
Immortalized by the Velvet
Underground song, *Venus in
Furs* tells the story of Severin
(Sacher-Masoch's thinly veiled
alter ego), whose only desire
is to become a sex slave to
his lover Wanda. With a bit of
coaxing, Wanda is persuaded
to don the furs and crack
the whip, and soon finds
she enjoys playing the cruel
mistress, much to Severin's
delight. Seen as a seminal
work of erotic fiction, *Venus
in Furs* remains *the* classic tale
of mistress and slave, with
plenty of genuinely erotic
passages in which Severin is
bound by Wanda's satin-clad
servants or left tied up at his
mistress's boots to endure
the cruel blows of her whip.
Things get a bit sticky at
the end when the game
takes an unexpected turn.
Severin ends up suffering
the humiliation of being
whipped by his mistress's
new lover, leading to a last-
minute change of heart
about their roles.

HiSTOiRE D'O/ THE STORY OF "O"

(Pauline Réage)
This French erotic novel
caused quite a stir when
first released in 1954. It's
an erotic fantasy about a
Parisian fashion model who
is trained to become sexually
objectified by her lover, and
subjected to a whole range
of humiliations including
whipping, incarceration, and
being used for sex by anyone
who desires her. The twist
comes about halfway into
the book, when the reader
discovers that "O" is perhaps
more willing than we were
first led to believe.

The Story of "O" was actually
written by respectable
scholar Anne Desclos, who
is said to have produced it
in response to her husband's
facetious remark one day that
"a woman couldn't write a
good erotic novel." Desclos
chose to keep her identity as
author a secret for 40 years
and, up until that point, many
critics claimed the book could
never have been written by
a woman.

Why the heroine is named
"O" remains open to debate.
It has been suggested that
"O" represents the ancient
symbol for the vagina, a
shorthand for "Object,"
or even the number zero,
suggesting that the heroine
of the story has surrendered
herself so completely that she
no longer really exists.

CLAIMING OF
SLEEPING BEAUTY
(A. N. Roquelaure)

Written under one of several *noms de plume* of author Ann Rice, the *Claiming of Sleeping Beauty* is highly erotic and well written. With its central theme being the tale of a woman's willing transformation into sexual submission, it's often described as a modern (and superior) version of *The Story of "O"*. Far from being naturalistic, the *Claiming of Sleeping Beauty* plays with fairytale imagery. It features dehumanized characters and a mythological fantasy world, an ideal playground, in fact, for Rice's erotically charged fetish fantasies. While some critics have read it as an allegory for the submissive role we all play in society, others have gone as far as to describe the message of the book as "the hell some women go through to satisfy their husband." Whether taken as genuine erotic fantasy or as a bitter social comment, it all lies in the maxim—one person's meat is another's poison.

LA NOUVELLE JUSTINE
(Marquis de Sade)

Justine remains de Sade's most famous work, and it was written in the Bastille during one of his many periods of incarceration. It's a vast and dense work of disturbing erotic fiction. It begins with the story of Justine, a young girl who, by denying the "truth" that God is evil, suffers an endless series of sexually depraved misfortunes. Then after several hundred pages, just as you think things can't get any more perverse, her evil sister turns up. . .

While most modern authors of fetish fiction are careful to acknowledge the distinction between fantasy and reality, de Sade was unashamed in his philosophy that "If you enjoy wickedness you should be wicked," making reading his literature more than a little uncomfortable at times. Even de Sade once raised an eyebrow at his own sadistic prose, however, declaring Justine to be "capable of corrupting the Devil."

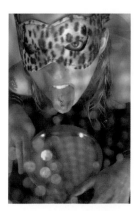

RESOURCE DIRECTORY

FETISH

PART EIGHT

RESOURCE DİRECTORY

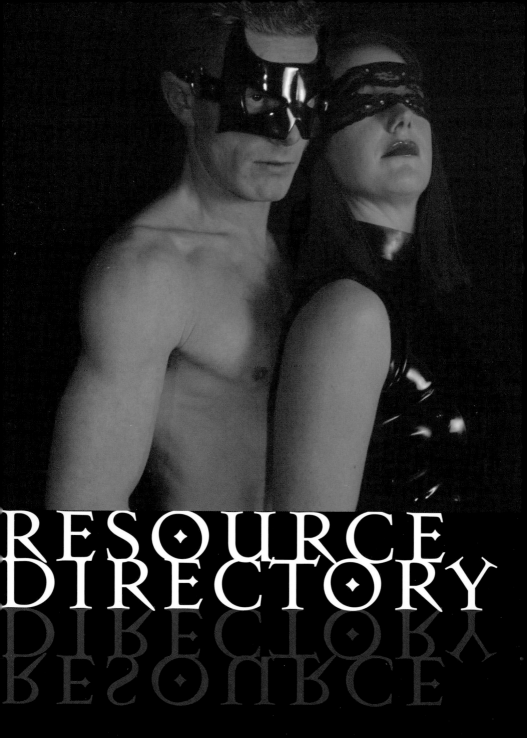

For those wishing to explore the world of fetish further, this chapter recommends good books, specialist websites, communities, online suppliers, magazines, clubs, and events through which to learn more, meet fellow perverts, and purchase those much sought-after kinky items.

Whatever your fancy—whether you're after spanking techniques, cross-dressing, pony play, or week-long kinky holidays in the Caribbean—you'll find a host of text, websites, communties, and events here.

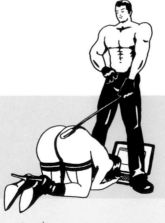

THE INTERNET IS A GATEWAY TO
MYRIAD FETISH COMMUNITIES

FETISH BOOKS

Art of Spanking
Milo Manaro

Come Hither: A Commonsense Guide to Kinky Sex
Gloria G. Brame

Consensual Sadomasochism
Bill Henkin and Sybil Holiday

Erotic Bondage Handbook
Jay Wiseman

Erotic Tickling
Michael Moran

Female Domination
Elise Sutton

The Fetish Fact Book
Paul Scott

Fetish, Fashion, Sex, and Power
Valerie Steele

Fetish Sex
Violet Blue and Thomas Roche

Sensuous Magic
Pat Califia

The Fine Art of Erotic Talk
Bonnie Gabriel

The Seductive Art of Japanese Bondage
Midori

The Tranny Guide
Vicky Lee

FETISH MAGAZINES

Bizarre

Marquis

Ritual

Secret

Skin Two

Taboo

Whiplash

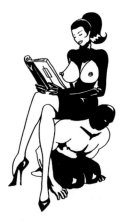

Online Fetish Suppliers

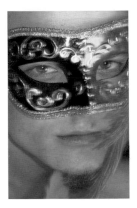

For suppliers of quality fetish clothing
and equipment, look no further than
the following online stores.

allheart.com (for genuine medical wear and equipment)

baroness.com

clubsissy.com (cross-dressing accessories)

costumes.org

cross-dress.com

demask.com

ebay.com (always a gamble but you can find some bargains!)

libidex.com

marquis.de (specializing in "heavy rubber")

medicaltoys.com

sexycostumes.com

skintwoclothing.com

stockroom.com (particularly good selection of fetish equipment)

thefantasygirl.com (cross-dressing accessories)

westwardbound.com

SPECIALIST SITES

FETISH SITES

bodyinflation.org

corset.dk

fingernailfetish.com

foot-fetish-planet.com

leatherdog.com
(many types of animal play
including dog training)

loonerz.com

maskon.com
(for mask-lovers)

messy-online.com
(wet/messy play)

myboobsite.com
(no description necessary)

pantyhosemama.com

sexy-midgets.com

thehumanequine.com
(pony play)

the-stampede.com
(pony play)

thumbsuckingadults.com
(human babies)

VIRTUAL COMMUNITIES

alt.com
(online dating for perverts)

collarme.com
(for meeting people into
the scene who are looking
to play. Also a good starting
point for finding out more
about different clubs, events,
and societies)

craigslist.org
(good for networking and
hooking up with other people
on the scene)

furnation.com
(website for the furry
community)

Munches
(These are informal
gatherings of like-minded
perverts who meet up to
chat, drink, share stories and
ideas, and that take place in
many cities around the world.
Check the Internet to see if
one exists near you. If not,
why not set up one yourself?)

tribe.net
(You'll find plenty of
communities and fetish-
related groups here)

EVENTS/CLUBS

blackandblueball.com
(New York)

clubslick.com
(San Francisco)

eros-guide.com/events
(fetish-related events in the
San Francisco Bay Area)

ffnto.com
(annual fetish weekend
in Toronto, Canada)

german-fetish-ball.com
(Germany)

hellfiresydney.com
(Australia)

kinkinthecaribbean.com
(week-long kinky event held
in Jamaica at Hedonism III)

skintworubberball.com
(annual UK fetish night and
one of the world's most
spectacular fetish events)

thefetishparty.com
(North America)

torturegarden.com
(the world's largest and most
famous fetish club)

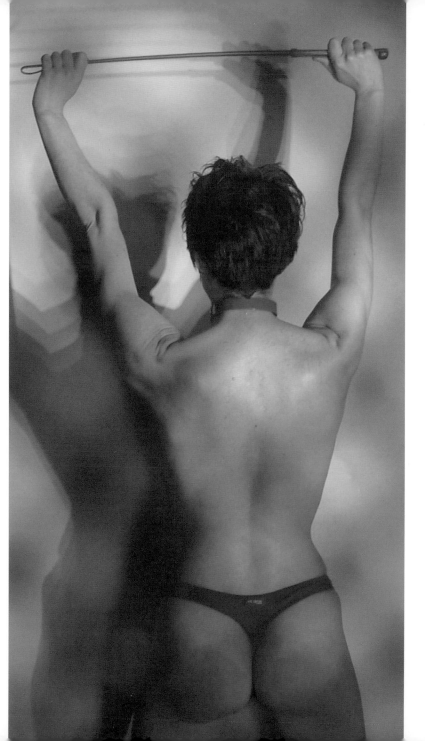

Index